THE OFFICIAL PATIENT'S SOURCEBOOK

on

THYROID CANCER

JAMES N. PARKER, M.D.
AND PHILIP M. PARKER, PH.D., EDITORS

ICON Health Publications
ICON Group International, Inc.
4370 La Jolla Village Drive, 4th Floor
San Diego, CA 92122 USA

Copyright ©2002 by ICON Group International, Inc.

Copyright ©2002 by ICON Group International, Inc. All rights reserved. This book is protected by copyright. No part of it may be reproduced, stored in a retrieval system, or transmitted in any form or by any means, dectronic, mechanical, photocopying, recording or otherwise, without written permission from the publisher.

Printed in the United States of America.

Last digit indicates print number: 10 9 8 7 6 4 5 3 2 1

Publisher, Health Care: Tiffany LaRochelle
Editor(s): James Parker, M.D., Philip Parker, Ph.D.

Publisher's note: The ideas, procedures, and suggestions contained in this book are not intended as a substitute for consultation with your physician. All matters regarding your health require medical supervision. As new medical or scientific information becomes available from academic and clinical research, recommended treatments and drug therapies may undergo changes. The authors, editors, and publisher have attempted to make the information in this book up to date and accurate in accord with accepted standards at the time of publication. The authors, editors, and publisher are not responsible for errors or omissions or for consequences from application of the book, and make no warranty, expressed or implied, in regard to the contents of this book. Any practice described in this book should be applied by the reader in accordance with professional standards of care used in regard to the unique circumstances that may apply in each situation, in close consultation with a qualified physician. The reader is advised to always check product information (package inserts) for changes and new information regarding dose and contraindications before taking any drug or pharmacological product. Caution is especially urged when using new or infrequently ordered drugs, herbal remedies, vitamins and supplements, alternative therapies, complementary therapies and medicines, and integrative medical treatments.

Cataloging-in-Publication Data

Parker, James N., 1961-
Parker, Philip M., 1960-

The Official Patient's Sourcebook on Thyroid Cancer: A Revised and Updated Directory for the Internet Age/James N. Parker and Philip M. Parker, editors
p.   cm.
Includes bibliographical references, glossary and index.
ISBN: 0-597-83489-X
1. Thyroid Cancer-Popular works.   I. Title.

Disclaimer

This publication is not intended to be used for the diagnosis or treatment of a health problem or as a substitute for consultation with licensed medical professionals. It is sold with the understanding that the publisher, editors, and authors are not engaging in the rendering of medical, psychological, financial, legal, or other professional services.

References to any entity, product, service, or source of information that may be contained in this publication should not be considered an endorsement, either direct or implied, by the publisher, editors or authors. ICON Group International, Inc., the editors, or the authors are not responsible for the content of any Web pages nor publications referenced in this publication.

Copyright Notice

If a physician wishes to copy limited passages from this sourcebook for patient use, this right is automatically granted without written permission from ICON Group International, Inc. (ICON Group). However, all of ICON Group publications are copyrighted. With exception to the above, copying our publications in whole or in part, for whatever reason, is a violation of copyright laws and can lead to penalties and fines. Should you want to copy tables, graphs or other materials, please contact us to request permission (e-mail: iconedit@san.rr.com). ICON Group often grants permission for very limited reproduction of our publications for internal use, press releases, and academic research. Such reproduction requires confirmed permission from ICON Group International Inc. **The disclaimer above must accompany all reproductions, in whole or in part, of this sourcebook.**

Dedication

To the healthcare professionals dedicating their time and efforts to the study of thyroid cancer.

Acknowledgements

The collective knowledge generated from academic and applied research summarized in various references has been critical in the creation of this sourcebook which is best viewed as a comprehensive compilation and collection of information prepared by various official agencies which directly or indirectly are dedicated to thyroid cancer. All of the *Official Patient's Sourcebooks* draw from various agencies and institutions associated with the United States Department of Health and Human Services, and in particular, the Office of the Secretary of Health and Human Services (OS), the Administration for Children and Families (ACF), the Administration on Aging (AOA), the Agency for Healthcare Research and Quality (AHRQ), the Agency for Toxic Substances and Disease Registry (ATSDR), the Centers for Disease Control and Prevention (CDC), the Food and Drug Administration (FDA), the Healthcare Financing Administration (HCFA), the Health Resources and Services Administration (HRSA), the Indian Health Service (IHS), the institutions of the National Institutes of Health (NIH), the Program Support Center (PSC), and the Substance Abuse and Mental Health Services Administration (SAMHSA). In addition to these sources, information gathered from the National Library of Medicine, the United States Patent Office, the European Union, and their related organizations has been invaluable in the creation of this sourcebook. Some of the work represented was financially supported by the Research and Development Committee at INSEAD. This support is gratefully acknowledged. Finally, special thanks are owed to Tiffany LaRochelle for her excellent editorial support.

About the Editors

James N. Parker, M.D.

Dr. James N. Parker received his Bachelor of Science degree in Psychobiology from the University of California, Riverside and his M.D. from the University of California, San Diego. In addition to authoring numerous research publications, he has lectured at various academic institutions. Dr. Parker is the medical editor for the *Official Patient's Sourcebook* series published by ICON Health Publications.

Philip M. Parker, Ph.D.

Philip M. Parker is the Eli Lilly Chair Professor of Innovation, Business and Society at INSEAD (Fontainebleau, France and Singapore). Dr. Parker has also been Professor at the University of California, San Diego and has taught courses at Harvard University, the Hong Kong University of Science and Technology, the Massachusetts Institute of Technology, Stanford University, and UCLA. Dr. Parker is the associate editor for the *Official Patient's Sourcebook* series published by ICON Health Publications.

About ICON Health Publications

In addition to thyroid cancer, *Official Patient's Sourcebooks* are available for the following related topics:

- The Official Patient's Sourcebook on Adrenocortical Carcinoma
- The Official Patient's Sourcebook on Islet Cell Carcinoma (endocrine Pancreas)
- The Official Patient's Sourcebook on Parathyroid Cancer
- The Official Patient's Sourcebook on Pheochromocytoma
- The Official Patient's Sourcebook on Pituitary Tumor

To discover more about ICON Health Publications, simply check with your preferred online booksellers, including Barnes & Noble.com and Amazon.com which currently carry all of our titles. Or, feel free to contact us directly for bulk purchases or institutional discounts:

ICON Group International, Inc.
4370 La Jolla Village Drive, Fourth Floor
San Diego, CA 92122 USA
Fax: 858-546-4341
Web site: **www.icongrouponline.com/health**

Table of Contents

INTRODUCTION 1
   Overview 1
   Organization 3
   Scope 3
   Moving Forward 4

PART I: THE ESSENTIALS 7

CHAPTER 1. THE ESSENTIALS ON THYROID CANCER: GUIDELINES 9
   Overview 9
   What Is Thyroid Cancer? 11
   Stages of Papillary Cancers of the Thyroid 12
   Stages of Follicular Cancers of the Thyroid 13
   Other Types or Stages of Thyroid Cancer 14
   How Is Thyroid Cancer Treated? 15
   Treatment by Stage 16
   To Learn More 19
   About PDQ 21
   More Guideline Sources 22
   Vocabulary Builder 26

CHAPTER 2. SEEKING GUIDANCE 29
   Overview 29
   Associations and Thyroid Cancer 29
   Cancer Support Groups 31
   The Cancer Information Service 33
   Finding Cancer Resources in Your Community 36
   Finding Doctors Who Specialize in Cancer Care 39
   Selecting Your Doctor 42
   Working with Your Doctor 43
   Finding a Cancer Treatment Facility 44
   Additional Cancer Support Information 46
   Vocabulary Builder 46

CHAPTER 3. CLINICAL TRIALS AND THYROID CANCER 49
   Overview 49
   Recent Trials on Thyroid Cancer 52
   Benefits and Risks 53
   Clinical Trials and Insurance Coverage 56
   Clinical Trials and Medicare Coverage 59
   Increasing the Likelihood of Insurance Coverage for Trials 60
   If Your Insurance Claim Is Denied after the Trial Has Begun 62
   Government Initiatives to Expand Insurance Coverage for Trials 65
   Keeping Current on Clinical Trials 66

General References 67
Vocabulary Builder 68

PART II: ADDITIONAL RESOURCES AND ADVANCED MATERIAL 73

CHAPTER 4. STUDIES ON THYROID CANCER 75
Overview 75
The Combined Health Information Database 75
Federally Funded Research on Thyroid Cancer 77
E-Journals: PubMed Central 89
The National Library of Medicine: PubMed 90
Vocabulary Builder 110

CHAPTER 5. BOOKS ON THYROID CANCER 117
Overview 117
Book Summaries: Federal Agencies 117
The National Library of Medicine Book Index 118
Chapters on Thyroid Cancer 122
General Home References 123
Vocabulary Builder 124

CHAPTER 6. MULTIMEDIA ON THYROID CANCER 127
Overview 127
Bibliography: Multimedia on Thyroid Cancer 127
Vocabulary Builder 130

CHAPTER 7. PERIODICALS AND NEWS ON THYROID CANCER 131
Overview 131
News Services & Press Releases 131
Newsletters on Thyroid Cancer 137
Newsletter Articles 138
Academic Periodicals Covering Thyroid Cancer 138
Vocabulary Builder 140

CHAPTER 8. PHYSICIAN GUIDELINES AND DATABASES 143
Overview 143
NIH Guidelines 143
What Is Thyroid Cancer? 144
Cellular Classification 146
Stage Information 147
TNM Definitions 147
AJCC Stage Groupings for Papillary or Follicular 148
AJCC Stage Groupings for Medullary 149
AJCC Stage Groupings for Undifferentiated (Anaplastic) 149
Papillary Staging 149
Follicular Staging 150
Medullary Staging 151

Anaplastic Staging 153
Treatment Option Overview 154
Stage I Papillary Thyroid Cancer 154
Stage I Follicular Thyroid Cancer 155
Stage II Papillary Thyroid Cancer 157
Stage II Follicular Thyroid Cancer 158
Stage III Papillary Thyroid Cancer 159
Stage III Follicular Thyroid Cancer 160
Stage IV Papillary Thyroid Cancer 160
Stage IV Follicular Thyroid Cancer 161
Medullary Thyroid Cancer 162
Anaplastic Thyroid Cancer 163
Recurrent Thyroid Cancer 164
NIH Databases 166
Other Commercial Databases 171
The Genome Project and Thyroid Cancer 171
Specialized References 176
Vocabulary Builder 177

CHAPTER 9. DISSERTATIONS ON THYROID CANCER 179
Overview 179
Dissertations on Thyroid Cancer 179
Keeping Current 180

PART III. APPENDICES 181

APPENDIX A. RESEARCHING YOUR MEDICATIONS 183
Overview 183
Your Medications: The Basics 184
Learning More about Your Medications 185
Commercial Databases 189
Drug Development and Approval 190
Understanding the Approval Process for New Cancer Drugs 191
The Role of the Federal Drug Administration (FDA) 192
Getting Drugs to Patients Who Need Them 195
Contraindications and Interactions (Hidden Dangers) 197
A Final Warning 199
General References 199
Vocabulary Builder 200

APPENDIX B. RESEARCHING ALTERNATIVE MEDICINE 201
Overview 201
What Is CAM? 202
What Are the Domains of Alternative Medicine? 203
Finding CAM References on Thyroid Cancer 208
Additional Web Resources 217
General References 221

APPENDIX C. FINDING MEDICAL LIBRARIES.................................225
Overview..*225*
Preparation *225*
Finding a Local Medical Library *226*
Medical Libraries Open to the Public....................................*226*
APPENDIX D. YOUR RIGHTS AND INSURANCE.............................233
Overview..*233*
Your Rights as a Patient..*233*
Patient Responsibilities *237*
Choosing an Insurance Plan...*238*
Medicare and Medicaid *240*
Financial Assistance for Cancer Care....................................*243*
NORD's Medication Assistance Programs *246*
Additional Resources...*247*
Vocabulary Builder...*247*

ONLINE GLOSSARIES 251
Online Dictionary Directories..*255*

THYROID CANCER GLOSSARY 257
General Dictionaries and Glossaries *275*

INDEX 278

INTRODUCTION

Overview

Dr. C. Everett Koop, former U.S. Surgeon General, once said, "The best prescription is knowledge."[1] The Agency for Healthcare Research and Quality (AHRQ) of the National Institutes of Health (NIH) echoes this view and recommends that every patient incorporate education into the treatment process. According to the AHRQ:

> Finding out more about your condition is a good place to start. By contacting groups that support your condition, visiting your local library, and searching on the Internet, you can find good information to help guide your treatment decisions. Some information may be hard to find — especially if you don't know where to look.[2]

As the AHRQ mentions, finding the right information is not an obvious task. Though many physicians and public officials had thought that the emergence of the Internet would do much to assist patients in obtaining reliable information, in March 2001 the National Institutes of Health issued the following warning:

> The number of Web sites offering health-related resources grows every day. Many sites provide valuable information, while others may have information that is unreliable or misleading.[3]

---

[1] Quotation from **http://www.drkoop.com**.
[2] The Agency for Healthcare Research and Quality (AHRQ): **http://www.ahcpr.gov/consumer/diaginfo.htm**.
[3] Adapted from the NIH, National Cancer Institute (NCI): **http://cancertrials.nci.nih.gov/beyond/evaluating.html**.

Since the late 1990s, physicians have seen a general increase in patient Internet usage rates. Patients frequently enter their doctor's offices with printed Web pages of home remedies in the guise of latest medical research. This scenario is so common that doctors often spend more time dispelling misleading information than guiding patients through sound therapies. *The Official Patient's Sourcebook on Thyroid Cancer* has been created for patients who have decided to make education and research an integral part of the treatment process. The pages that follow will tell you where and how to look for information covering virtually all topics related to thyroid cancer, from the essentials to the most advanced areas of research.

The title of this book includes the word "official." This reflects the fact that the sourcebook draws from public, academic, government, and peer-reviewed research. Selected readings from various agencies are reproduced to give you some of the latest official information available to date on thyroid cancer.

Given patients' increasing sophistication in using the Internet, abundant references to reliable Internet-based resources are provided throughout this sourcebook. Where possible, guidance is provided on how to obtain free-of-charge, primary research results as well as more detailed information via the Internet. E-book and electronic versions of this sourcebook are fully interactive with each of the Internet sites mentioned (clicking on a hyperlink automatically opens your browser to the site indicated). Hard copy users of this sourcebook can type cited Web addresses directly into their browsers to obtain access to the corresponding sites. Since we are working with ICON Health Publications, hard copy *Sourcebooks* are frequently updated and printed on demand to ensure that the information provided is current.

In addition to extensive references accessible via the Internet, every chapter presents a "Vocabulary Builder." Many health guides offer glossaries of technical or uncommon terms in an appendix. In editing this sourcebook, we have decided to place a smaller glossary within each chapter that covers terms used in that chapter. Given the technical nature of some chapters, you may need to revisit many sections. Building one's vocabulary of medical terms in such a gradual manner has been shown to improve the learning process.

We must emphasize that no sourcebook on thyroid cancer should affirm that a specific diagnostic procedure or treatment discussed in a research study, patent, or doctoral dissertation is "correct" or your best option. This sourcebook is no exception. Each patient is unique. Deciding on appropriate options is always up to the patient in consultation with their physician and healthcare providers.

Organization

This sourcebook is organized into three parts. Part I explores basic techniques to researching thyroid cancer (e.g. finding guidelines on diagnosis, treatments, and prognosis), followed by a number of topics, including information on how to get in touch with organizations, associations, or other patient networks dedicated to thyroid cancer. It also gives you sources of information that can help you find a doctor in your local area specializing in treating thyroid cancer. Collectively, the material presented in Part I is a complete primer on basic research topics for patients with thyroid cancer.

Part II moves on to advanced research dedicated to thyroid cancer. Part II is intended for those willing to invest many hours of hard work and study. It is here that we direct you to the latest scientific and applied research on thyroid cancer. When possible, contact names, links via the Internet, and summaries are provided. It is in Part II where the vocabulary process becomes important as authors publishing advanced research frequently use highly specialized language. In general, every attempt is made to recommend "free-to-use" options.

Part III provides appendices of useful background reading for all patients with thyroid cancer or related disorders. The appendices are dedicated to more pragmatic issues faced by many patients with thyroid cancer. Accessing materials via medical libraries may be the only option for some readers, so a guide is provided for finding local medical libraries which are open to the public. Part III, therefore, focuses on advice that goes beyond the biological and scientific issues facing patients with thyroid cancer.

Scope

While this sourcebook covers thyroid cancer, your doctor, research publications, and specialists may refer to your condition using a variety of terms. Therefore, you should understand that thyroid cancer is often considered a synonym or a condition closely related to the following:

- Lymphoma
- Mediastinal Lymphadenopathy

4 Thyroid Cancer

- Mediastinal Mass
- Neurogenic Tumors
- Teratoma
- Thymoma
- Thyroid Tumor

In addition to synonyms and related conditions, physicians may refer to thyroid cancer using certain coding systems. The International Classification of Diseases, 9th Revision, Clinical Modification (ICD-9-CM) is the most commonly used system of classification for the world's illnesses. Your physician may use this coding system as an administrative or tracking tool. The following classification is commonly used for thyroid cancer:[4]

- 161.3 laryngeal cartilages
- 193 malignant neoplasm of thyroid gland
- 212.1 larynx
- 226 benign neoplasm of thyroid glands

For the purposes of this sourcebook, we have attempted to be as inclusive as possible, looking for official information for all of the synonyms relevant to thyroid cancer. You may find it useful to refer to synonyms when accessing databases or interacting with healthcare professionals and medical librarians.

Moving Forward

Since the 1980s, the world has seen a proliferation of healthcare guides covering most illnesses. Some are written by patients or their family members. These generally take a layperson's approach to understanding and coping with an illness or disorder. They can be uplifting, encouraging, and highly supportive. Other guides are authored by physicians or other healthcare providers who have a more clinical outlook. Each of these two styles of guide has its purpose and can be quite useful.

As editors, we have chosen a third route. We have chosen to expose you to as many sources of official and peer-reviewed information as practical, for

---

[4] This list is based on the official version of the World Health Organization's 9th Revision, International Classification of Diseases (ICD-9). According to the National Technical Information Service, "ICD-9CM extensions, interpretations, modifications, addenda, or errata other than those approved by the U.S. Public Health Service and the Health Care Financing Administration are not to be considered official and should not be utilized. Continuous maintenance of the ICD-9-CM is the responsibility of the federal government."

the purpose of educating you about basic and advanced knowledge as recognized by medical science today. You can think of this sourcebook as your personal Internet age reference librarian.

Why "Internet age"? All too often, patients diagnosed with thyroid cancer will log on to the Internet, type words into a search engine, and receive several Web site listings which are mostly irrelevant or redundant. These patients are left to wonder where the relevant information is, and how to obtain it. Since only the smallest fraction of information dealing with thyroid cancer is even indexed in search engines, a non-systematic approach often leads to frustration and disappointment. With this sourcebook, we hope to direct you to the information you need that you would not likely find using popular Web directories. Beyond Web listings, in many cases we will reproduce brief summaries or abstracts of available reference materials. These abstracts often contain distilled information on topics of discussion.

While we focus on the more scientific aspects of thyroid cancer, there is, of course, the emotional side to consider. Later in the sourcebook, we provide a chapter dedicated to helping you find peer groups and associations that can provide additional support beyond research produced by medical science. We hope that the choices we have made give you the most options available in moving forward. In this way, we wish you the best in your efforts to incorporate this educational approach into your treatment plan.

The Editors

PART I: THE ESSENTIALS

ABOUT PART I

Part I has been edited to give you access to what we feel are "the essentials" on thyroid cancer. The essentials of a disease typically include the definition or description of the disease, a discussion of who it affects, the signs or symptoms associated with the disease, tests or diagnostic procedures that might be specific to the disease, and treatments for the disease. Your doctor or healthcare provider may have already explained the essentials of thyroid cancer to you or even given you a pamphlet or brochure describing thyroid cancer. Now you are searching for more in-depth information. As editors, we have decided, nevertheless, to include a discussion on where to find essential information that can complement what your doctor has already told you. In this section we recommend a process, not a particular Web site or reference book. The process ensures that, as you search the Web, you gain background information in such a way as to maximize your understanding.

CHAPTER 1. THE ESSENTIALS ON THYROID CANCER: GUIDELINES

Overview

Official agencies, as well as federally funded institutions supported by national grants, frequently publish a variety of guidelines on thyroid cancer. These are typically called "Fact Sheets" or "Guidelines." They can take the form of a brochure, information kit, pamphlet, or flyer. Often they are only a few pages in length. The great advantage of guidelines over other sources is that they are often written with the patient in mind. Since new guidelines on thyroid cancer can appear at any moment and be published by a number of sources, the best approach to finding guidelines is to systematically scan the Internet-based services that post them.

The National Institutes of Health (NIH)[5]

The National Institutes of Health (NIH) is the first place to search for relatively current patient guidelines and fact sheets on thyroid cancer. Originally founded in 1887, the NIH is one of the world's foremost medical research centers and the federal focal point for medical research in the United States. At any given time, the NIH supports some 35,000 research grants at universities, medical schools, and other research and training institutions, both nationally and internationally. The rosters of those who have conducted research or who have received NIH support over the years include the world's most illustrious scientists and physicians. Among them are 97 scientists who have won the Nobel Prize for achievement in medicine.

---

[5] Adapted from the NIH: **http://www.nih.gov/about/NIHoverview.html**.

10 Thyroid Cancer

There is no guarantee that any one Institute will have a guideline on a specific disease, though the National Institutes of Health collectively publish over 600 guidelines for both common and rare diseases. The best way to access NIH guidelines is via the Internet. Although the NIH is organized into many different Institutes and Offices, the following is a list of key Web sites where you are most likely to find NIH clinical guidelines and publications dealing with thyroid cancer and associated conditions:

- Office of the Director (OD); guidelines consolidated across agencies available at **http://www.nih.gov/health/consumer/conkey.htm**

- National Library of Medicine (NLM); extensive encyclopedia (A.D.A.M., Inc.) with guidelines available at **http://www.nlm.nih.gov/medlineplus/healthtopics.html**

- National Cancer Institute (NCI); guidelines available at **http://cancernet.nci.nih.gov/pdq/pdq_treatment.shtml**

Among the above, the National Cancer Institute (NCI) is particularly noteworthy. The NCI coordinates the National Cancer Program, which conducts and supports research, training, health information dissemination, and other programs with respect to the cause, diagnosis, prevention, and treatment of cancer, rehabilitation from cancer, and the continuing care of cancer patients and the families of cancer patients.[6] Specifically, the Institute:

- Supports and coordinates research projects conducted by universities, hospitals, research foundations, and businesses throughout this country and abroad through research grants and cooperative agreements.

- Conducts research in its own laboratories and clinics.

- Supports education and training in fundamental sciences and clinical disciplines for participation in basic and clinical research programs and treatment programs relating to cancer through career awards, training grants, and fellowships.

- Supports research projects in cancer control.

- Supports a national network of cancer centers.

- Collaborates with voluntary organizations and other national and foreign institutions engaged in cancer research and training activities.

- Encourages and coordinates cancer research by industrial concerns where such concerns evidence a particular capability for programmatic research.

- Collects and disseminates information on cancer.

---

[6] This paragraph has been adapted from the NCI: **http://www.nci.nih.gov/**. "Adapted" signifies that a passage has been reproduced exactly or slightly edited for this book.

- Supports construction of laboratories, clinics, and related facilities necessary for cancer research through the award of construction grants.

The NCI, established under the National Cancer Act of 1937, is the Federal Government's principal agency for cancer research and training. The National Cancer Act of 1971 broadened the scope and responsibilities of the NCI and created the National Cancer Program. Over the years, legislative amendments have maintained the NCI authorities and responsibilities and added new information dissemination mandates as well as a requirement to assess the incorporation of state-of-the-art cancer treatments into clinical practice. Information dissemination is made possible through the NCI Online at **www.cancer.gov**. Cancer.gov offers to the public and physicians up-to-date information on the latest cancer research, current and upcoming clinical trials, statistics, research programs, and research funding.

The following patient guideline was recently published by the NCI on thyroid cancer.

What Is Thyroid Cancer?[7]

Cancer of the thyroid is a disease in which cancer (malignant) cells are found in the tissues of the thyroid gland. The thyroid gland is at the base of the throat. It has two lobes, one on the right side and one on the left. The thyroid gland makes important hormones that help the body function normally.

Cancer of the thyroid is more common in women than in men. Most patients are between 25 and 65 years old. People who have been exposed to large amounts of radiation, or who have had radiation treatment for medical problems in the head and neck have a higher chance of getting thyroid cancer. The cancer may not occur until 20 years or longer after radiation treatment.

A doctor should be seen if there is a lump or swelling in the front of the neck or in other parts of the neck.

If there are symptoms, a doctor will feel the patient's thyroid and check for lumps in the neck. The doctor may order blood tests and special scans to see whether a lump in the thyroid is making too many hormones. The doctor may want to take a small amount of tissue from the thyroid. This is called a

---

[7] The following guidelines appeared on the NCI website on Aug. 26, 2002. The text was last modified in August 2002. The text has been adapted for this sourcebook.

biopsy. To do this, a small needle is inserted into the thyroid at the base of the throat and some tissue is drawn out. The tissue is then looked at under a microscope to see whether it contains cancer.

There are four main types of cancer of the thyroid (based on how the cancer cells look under a microscope): papillary, follicular, medullary, and anaplastic. The chance of recovery (prognosis) depends on the type of thyroid cancer, whether it is just in the thyroid or has spread to other parts of the body (stage), and the patient's age and overall health. Some types of thyroid cancer grow much faster than others.

The genes in our cells carry the hereditary information from our parents. An abnormal gene has been found in patients with some forms of thyroid cancer. If medullary thyroid cancer is found, the patient may have been born with a certain abnormal gene which may have led to the cancer. Family members may have also inherited this abnormal gene. Tests have been developed to determine who has the genetic defect long before any cancer appears. It is important that the patient and his or her family members (children, grandchildren, parents, brothers, sisters, nieces and nephews) see a doctor about tests that will show if the abnormal gene is present. These tests are confidential and can help the doctor help patients. Family members, including young children, who don't have cancer, but do have this abnormal gene, may reduce the chance of developing medullary thyroid cancer by having surgery to safely remove the thyroid gland (thyroidectomy).

Stages of Papillary Cancers of the Thyroid

Once cancer of the thyroid is found (diagnosed), more tests will be done to find out if cancer cells have spread to other parts of the body. This is called staging. A doctor needs to know the stage of the disease to plan treatment.

The following stages are used for papillary cancers of the thyroid:

Stage I Papillary

Cancer is only in the thyroid and may be found in one or both lobes.

Stage II Papillary

In patients younger than 45 years of age:
- Cancer has spread beyond the thyroid.

In patients older than 45 years of age:
- Cancer is only in the thyroid and larger than 1 centimeter (about 1/2 inch).

Stage III Papillary

Cancer is found in patients older than 45 years of age and has spread outside the thyroid (but not outside of the neck) or has spread to the lymph nodes.

Stage IV Papillary

Cancer is found in patients older than 45 years of age and has spread to other parts of the body, such as the lungs and bones.

Stages of Follicular Cancers of the Thyroid

The following stages are used for follicular cancers of the thyroid:

Stage I Follicular

Cancer is only in the thyroid and may be found in one or both lobes.

Stage II Follicular

In patients younger than 45 years of age:
- Cancer has spread beyond the thyroid.

In patients older than 45 years of age:
- Cancer is only in the thyroid and larger than 1 centimeter (about 1/2 inch).

Stage III Follicular

Cancer is found in patients older than 45 years of age and has spread outside the thyroid (but not outside of the neck) or to the lymph nodes.

Stage IV Follicular

Cancer is found in patients older than 45 years of age and has spread to other parts of the body, such as the lungs and bones.

Other Types or Stages of Thyroid Cancer

Other types or stages of thyroid cancer include the following:

Stage I Medullary

Cancer is less than 1 centimeter (about 1/2 inch) in size.

Stage II Medullary

Cancer is between 1 and 4 centimeters (about 1/2 to 1 1/2 inches) in size.

Stage III Medullary

Cancer has spread to the lymph nodes.

Stage IV Medullary

Cancer has spread to other parts of the body.

Anaplastic

There is no staging system for anaplastic cancer of the thyroid. This type of cancer of the thyroid grows faster than the other types.

Recurrent

Recurrent disease means that the cancer has come back (recurred) after it has been treated. It may come back in the thyroid or in another part of the body.

How Is Thyroid Cancer Treated?

There are treatments for all patients with cancer of the thyroid. Four types of treatment are used:

- Surgery (taking out the cancer)
- Radiation therapy (using high-dose x-rays or other high-energy rays to kill cancer cells)
- Hormone therapy (using hormones to stop cancer cells from growing)
- Chemotherapy (using drugs to kill cancer cells)

Surgery

Surgery is the most common treatment of cancer of the thyroid. A doctor may remove the cancer using one of the following operations:

- Lobectomy removes only the side of the thyroid where the cancer is found. Lymph nodes in the area may be taken out (biopsied) to see if they contain cancer.
- Near-total thyroidectomy removes all of the thyroid except for a small part.
- Total thyroidectomy removes the entire thyroid.
- Lymph node dissection removes lymph nodes in the neck that contain cancer.

Radiation Therapy

Radiation therapy uses high-energy x-rays to kill cancer cells and shrink tumors. Radiation for cancer of the thyroid may come from a machine outside the body (external radiation therapy) or from drinking a liquid that contains radioactive iodine. Because the thyroid takes up iodine, the radioactive iodine collects in any thyroid tissue remaining in the body and kills the cancer cells.

Hormone Therapy

Hormone therapy uses hormones to stop cancer cells from growing. In treating cancer of the thyroid, hormones can be used to stop the body from making other hormones that might make cancer cells grow. Hormones are usually given as pills.

Chemotherapy

Chemotherapy uses drugs to kill cancer cells. Chemotherapy may be taken by pill, or it may be put into the body by a needle in the vein or muscle. Chemotherapy is called a systemic treatment because the drug enters the bloodstream, travels through the body, and can kill cancer cells outside the thyroid.

Treatment by Stage

Treatment of cancer of the thyroid depends on the type and stage of the disease, and the patient's age and overall health.

Standard treatment may be considered because of its effectiveness in patients in past studies, or participation in a clinical trial may be considered. Not all patients are cured with standard therapy and some standard treatments may have more side effects than are desired. For these reasons, clinical trials are designed to find better ways to treat cancer patients and are based on the most up-to-date information. Clinical trials are ongoing in many parts of the country for some patients with cancer of the thyroid. To learn more about clinical trials, call the Cancer Information Service at 1-800-4-CANCER (1-800-422-6237); TTY at 1-800-332-8615.

Stage I Papillary Thyroid Cancer

Treatment may be one of the following:

- Surgery to remove one lobe of the thyroid (lobectomy), followed by hormone therapy. Radioactive iodine also may be given following surgery.
- Surgery to remove the thyroid (total thyroidectomy).

Stage I Follicular Thyroid Cancer

Treatment may be one of the following:

- Surgery to remove the thyroid (total thyroidectomy).
- Surgery to remove one lobe of the thyroid (lobectomy), followed by hormone therapy. Radioactive iodine also may be given following surgery.

Stage II Papillary Thyroid Cancer

Treatment may be one of the following:

- Surgery to remove one lobe of the thyroid (lobectomy) and lymph nodes that contain cancer, followed by hormone therapy. Radioactive iodine also may be given following surgery.
- Surgery to remove the thyroid (total thyroidectomy).

Stage II Follicular Thyroid Cancer

Treatment may be one of the following:

- Surgery to remove the thyroid (total thyroidectomy).
- Surgery to remove one lobe of the thyroid (lobectomy) and lymph nodes that contain cancer, followed by hormone therapy. Radioactive iodine also may be given following surgery.

Stage III Papillary Thyroid Cancer

Treatment may be one of the following:

- Surgery to remove the entire thyroid (total thyroidectomy) and lymph nodes where cancer has spread.
- Total thyroidectomy followed by radiation therapy with radioactive iodine or external beam radiation therapy.

Stage III Follicular Thyroid Cancer

Treatment may be one of the following:

- Surgery to remove the entire thyroid (total thyroidectomy) and lymph nodes or other tissues around the thyroid where the cancer has spread.
- Total thyroidectomy followed by radioactive iodine or external beam radiation therapy.

Stage IV Papillary Thyroid Cancer

Treatment may be one of the following:

- Radioactive iodine.
- External beam radiation therapy.
- Hormone therapy.
- A clinical trial of chemotherapy.

Stage IV Follicular Thyroid Cancer

Treatment may be one of the following:

- Radioactive iodine.
- External beam radiation therapy.
- Hormone therapy.
- A clinical trial of chemotherapy.

Medullary Thyroid Cancer

Treatment will probably be surgery to remove the entire thyroid (total thyroidectomy) unless the cancer has spread to other parts of the body. If lymph nodes in the neck contain cancer, the lymph nodes in the neck will be removed (lymph node dissection). If the cancer has spread to other parts of the body, chemotherapy may be given.

Anaplastic Thyroid Cancer

Treatment may be one of the following:

- Surgery to remove the thyroid and the tissues around it. Because this cancer often spreads very quickly to other tissues, a doctor may have to take out part of the tube through which a person breathes. The doctor will then make an airway in the throat so the patient can breathe. This is called a tracheostomy.
- Total thyroidectomy to reduce symptoms if the disease remains in the area of the thyroid.
- External beam radiation therapy.
- Chemotherapy.
- Clinical trials studying new methods of treatment of thyroid cancer.

Recurrent Thyroid Cancer

The choice of treatment depends on the type of thyroid cancer the patient has, the kind of treatment the patient had before, and where the cancer comes back. Treatment may be one of the following:

- Surgery with or without radioactive iodine.
- External beam radiation therapy to relieve symptoms caused by the cancer.
- Chemotherapy.
- Radioactive iodine.
- Radiation therapy given during surgery.
- Clinical trials.

To Learn More

Call

For more information, U.S. residents may call the National Cancer Institute's (NCI's) Cancer Information Service toll-free at 1-800-4-CANCER (1-800-422-6237), Monday through Friday from 9:00 a.m. to 4:30 p.m. Deaf and hard-of-hearing callers with TTY equipment may call 1-800-332-8615. The call is free and a trained Cancer Information Specialist is available to answer your questions.

Web Sites and Organizations

The NCI's Cancer.gov Web site (**http://cancer.gov**) provides online access to information on cancer, clinical trials, and other Web sites and organizations that offer support and resources for cancer patients and their families. There are also many other places where people can get materials and information about cancer treatment and services. Local hospitals may have information on local and regional agencies that offer information about finances, getting to and from treatment, receiving care at home, and dealing with problems associated with cancer treatment.

Publications

The NCI has booklets and other materials for patients, health professionals, and the public. These publications discuss types of cancer, methods of cancer treatment, coping with cancer, and clinical trials. Some publications provide information on tests for cancer, cancer causes and prevention, cancer statistics, and NCI research activities. NCI materials on these and other topics may be ordered online or printed directly from the NCI Publications Locator (**https://cissecure.nci.nih.gov/ncipubs**). These materials can also be ordered by telephone from the Cancer Information Service toll-free at 1-800-4-CANCER (1-800-422-6237), TTY at 1-800-332-8615.

LiveHelp

The NCI's LiveHelp service, a program available on several of the Institute's Web sites, provides Internet users with the ability to chat online with an Information Specialist. The service is available from Monday - Friday 9:00 AM - 10:00 PM Eastern Time. Information Specialists can help Internet users find information on NCI Web sites and answer questions about cancer.

Write

For more information from the NCI, please write to this address:

National Cancer Institute
Office of Communications
31 Center Drive, MSC 2580
Bethesda, MD 20892-2580

About PDQ

PDQ Is a Comprehensive Cancer Database Available on Cancer.gov

PDQ is the National Cancer Institute's (NCI's) comprehensive cancer information database. Most of the information contained in PDQ is available online at Cancer.gov (**http://cancer.gov**), the NCI's Web site. PDQ is provided as a service of the NCI. The NCI is part of the National Institutes of Health, the federal government's focal point for biomedical research.

PDQ Contains Cancer Information Summaries

The PDQ database contains summaries of the latest published information on cancer prevention, detection, genetics, treatment, supportive care, and complementary and alternative medicine. Most summaries are available in two versions. The health professional versions provide detailed information written in technical language. The patient versions are written in easy-to-understand, non-technical language. Both versions provide current and accurate cancer information.

The PDQ cancer information summaries are developed by cancer experts and reviewed regularly. Editorial Boards made up of experts in oncology and related specialties are responsible for writing and maintaining the cancer information summaries. The summaries are reviewed regularly and changes are made as new information becomes available. The date on each summary ("Date Last Modified") indicates the time of the most recent change.

PDQ Contains Information on Clinical Trials

Before starting treatment, patients may want to think about taking part in a clinical trial. A clinical trial is a study to answer a scientific question, such as whether one treatment is better than another. Trials are based on past studies and what has been learned in the laboratory. Each trial answers certain scientific questions in order to find new and better ways to help cancer patients. During treatment clinical trials, information is collected about new treatments, the risks involved, and how well they do or do not work. If a clinical trial shows that a new treatment is better than one currently being used, the new treatment may become "standard."

Listings of clinical trials are included in PDQ and are available online at Cancer.gov (**http://cancer.gov/clinical_trials**). Descriptions of the trials are available in health professional and patient versions. Many cancer doctors who take part in clinical trials are also listed in PDQ. For more information, call the Cancer Information Service at 1-800-4-CANCER (1-800-422-6237); TTY at 1-800-332-8615.

More Guideline Sources

The guideline above on thyroid cancer is only one example of the kind of material that you can find online and free of charge. The remainder of this chapter will direct you to other sources which either publish or can help you find additional guidelines on topics related to thyroid cancer. Many of the guidelines listed below address topics that may be of particular relevance to your specific situation or of special interest to only some patients with thyroid cancer. Due to space limitations these sources are listed in a concise manner. Do not hesitate to consult the following sources by either using the Internet hyperlink provided, or, in cases where the contact information is provided, contacting the publisher or author directly.

Topic Pages: MEDLINEplus

For patients wishing to go beyond guidelines published by specific Institutes of the NIH, the National Library of Medicine has created a vast and patient-oriented healthcare information portal called MEDLINEplus. Within this Internet-based system are "health topic pages." You can think of a health topic page as a guide to patient guides. To access this system, log on to **http://www.nlm.nih.gov/medlineplus/healthtopics.html**.

If you do not find topics of interest when browsing health topic pages, then you can choose to use the advanced search utility of MEDLINEplus at **http://www.nlm.nih.gov/medlineplus/advancedsearch.html**. This utility is similar to the NIH Search Utility, with the exception that it only includes material linked within the MEDLINEplus system (mostly patient-oriented information). It also has the disadvantage of generating unstructured results. We recommend, therefore, that you use this method only if you have a very targeted search.

The Combined Health Information Database (CHID)

CHID Online is a reference tool that maintains a database directory of thousands of journal articles and patient education guidelines on thyroid cancer and related conditions. One of the advantages of CHID over other sources is that it offers summaries that describe the guidelines available, including contact information and pricing. CHID's general Web site is **http://chid.nih.gov/**. To search this database, go to **http://chid.nih.gov/detail/detail.html**. In particular, you can use the advanced search options to look up pamphlets, reports, brochures, and information kits. The following was recently posted in this archive:

- **Thyroid Disease in the Elderly**

  Source: Boston, MA: Thyroid Foundation of America, Inc. 1994. [10 p.].

  Contact: Available from Thyroid Foundation of America Inc. Ruth Sleeper Hall, Room 350, 40 Parkman Street, Boston, MA 02114-2698. (800) 832-8321 or (617) 726-8500; FAX (617) 726-4136.

  Summary: This brochure discusses hyperthyroidism and hypothyroidism in patients over the age of 60. Specific information is presented about symptoms, diagnosis, treatment, and drug therapies for each of these conditions. Diagnosis and treatment of thyroid nodules and thyroid cancer in older people are also discussed.

- **Childhood Head and Neck Irradiation**

  Source: Boston, MA: Thyroid Foundation of America, Inc. December 1993. [6 p.].

  Contact: Available from Thyroid Foundation of America Inc. Ruth Sleeper Hall, Room 350, 40 Parkman Street, Boston, MA 02114-2698. (800) 832-8321, (617) 726-8500; FAX (617) 726-4136.

  Summary: This brochure is intended for persons who recieved head and neck irradiation during infancy and childhood. The relationship between early irradiation and thyroid cancer is examined, and the process of confirming x-ray exposure during childhood is discussed. Additional topics include diagnosing possible thyroid disorders due to past irradiation, the use of thyroid hormone medication, and the importance of regular annual examinations.

- **Cancer of the Thyroid: Papillary and Follicular Thyroid Cancer**

    Source: Boston, MA: Thyroid Foundation of America, Inc. 1994. [10 p.].

    Contact: Available from Thyroid Foundation of America Inc. Ruth Sleeper Hall, Room 350, 40 Parkman Street, Boston, MA 02114-2698. (800) 832-8321, (617) 726-8500; FAX (617) 726-4136.

    Summary: This brochure discusses the most common types of thyroid tumors. Specific information is presented about the symptoms, characteristics, diagnosis, and treatment of papillary thyroid cancer and follicular thyroid carcinoma, including the use of radioiodine therapy. The importance of periodic follow-up examinations and thyroid hormone treatment is also discussed.

The National Guideline Clearinghouse™

The National Guideline Clearinghouse™ offers hundreds of evidence-based clinical practice guidelines published in the United States and other countries. You can search their site located at **http://www.guideline.gov** by using the keyword "thyroid cancer" or synonyms. The following was recently posted:

- **Procedure guideline for extended scintigraphy for differentiated thyroid cancer.**

    Source: Society of Nuclear Medicine, Inc..; 1999 February; 15 pages

    http://www.guideline.gov/FRAMESETS/guideline_fs.asp?guideline=000621&sSearch_string=thyroid+cancer

Healthfinder™

Healthfinder™ is an additional source sponsored by the U.S. Department of Health and Human Services which offers links to hundreds of other sites that contain healthcare information. This Web site is located at **http://www.healthfinder.gov**. Again, keyword searches can be used to find guidelines. The following was recently found in this database:

- **Frequently Asked Questions on Potassium Iodide (KI)**

    Summary: Answers frequently asked questions about potassium iodide as a preventive measure for thyroid cancer from radiation exposure.

    Source: Center for Drug Evaluation and Research, U.S. Food and Drug Administration

    http://www.healthfinder.gov/scripts/recordpass.asp?RecordType=0&RecordID=6698

The NIH Search Utility

After browsing the references listed at the beginning of this chapter, you may want to explore the NIH Search Utility. This allows you to search for documents on over 100 selected Web sites that comprise the NIH-WEB-SPACE. Each of these servers is "crawled" and indexed on an ongoing basis. Your search will produce a list of various documents, all of which will relate in some way to thyroid cancer. The drawbacks of this approach are that the information is not organized by theme and that the references are often a mix of information for professionals and patients. Nevertheless, a large number of the listed Web sites provide useful background information. We can only recommend this route, therefore, for relatively rare or specific disorders, or when using highly targeted searches. To use the NIH search utility, visit the following Web page: **http://search.nih.gov/index.html**.

Additional Web Sources

A number of Web sites that often link to government sites are available to the public. These can also point you in the direction of essential information. The following is a representative sample:

- AOL: **http://search.aol.com/cat.adp?id=168&layer=&from=subcats**
- drkoop.com®: **http://www.drkoop.com/conditions/ency/index.html**
- Family Village: **http://www.familyvillage.wisc.edu/specific.htm**
- Google: **http://directory.google.com/Top/Health/Conditions_and_Diseases/**
- Med Help International: **http://www.medhelp.org/HealthTopics/A.html**
- Open Directory Project: **http://dmoz.org/Health/Conditions_and_Diseases/**
- Yahoo.com: **http://dir.yahoo.com/Health/Diseases_and_Conditions/**

- WebMD®Health: **http://my.webmd.com/health_topics**

Vocabulary Builder

The material in this chapter may have contained a number of unfamiliar words. The following Vocabulary Builder introduces you to terms used in this chapter that have not been covered in the previous chapter:

Anaplastic: A term used to describe cancer cells that divide rapidly and bear little or no resemblance to normal cells. [NIH]

Biopsy: The removal of cells or tissues for examination under a microscope. When only a sample of tissue is removed, the procedure is called an incisional biopsy or core biopsy. When an entire tumor or lesion is removed, the procedure is called an excisional biopsy. When a sample of tissue or fluid is removed with a needle, the procedure is called a needle biopsy or fine-needle aspiration. [NIH]

Carcinoma: Cancer that begins in the skin or in tissues that line or cover internal organs. [NIH]

Cell: The individual unit that makes up all of the tissues of the body. All living things are made up of one or more cells. [NIH]

Chemotherapy: Treatment with anticancer drugs. [NIH]

Gene: The functional and physical unit of heredity passed from parent to offspring. Genes are pieces of DNA, and most genes contain the information for making a specific protein. [NIH]

Gland: An organ that produces and releases one or more substances for use in the body. Some glands produce fluids that affect tissues or organs. Others produce hormones or participate in blood production. [NIH]

Hormones: Chemicals produced by glands in the body and circulated in the bloodstream. Hormones control the actions of certain cells or organs. [NIH]

Hyperthyroidism: A condition in which the thyroid gland produces too much thyroid hormone. [NIH]

Hypothyroidism: Deficiency of thyroid activity. In adults, it is most common in women and is characterized by decrease in basal metabolic rate, tiredness and lethargy, sensitivity to cold, and menstrual disturbances. If untreated, it progresses to full-blown myxoedema. In infants, severe hypothyroidism leads to cretinism. In juveniles, the manifestations are intermediate, with less severe mental and developmental retardation and only mild symptoms of the adult form. When due to pituitary deficiency of thyrotropin secretion it is called secondary hypothyroidism. [EU]

Iodine: A nonmetallic element of the halogen group that is represented by the atomic symbol I, atomic number 53, and atomic weight of 126.90. It is a nutritionally essential element, especially important in thyroid hormone synthesis. In solution, it has anti-infective properties and is used topically. [NIH]

Lobe: A portion of an organ such as the liver, lung, breast, or brain. [NIH]

Lobectomy: The removal of a lobe. [NIH]

Lymph: The almost colorless fluid that travels through the lymphatic system and carries cells that help fight infection and disease. [NIH]

Lymphoma: Cancer that arises in cells of the lymphatic system. [NIH]

Malignant: Cancerous; a growth with a tendency to invade and destroy nearby tissue and spread to other parts of the body. [NIH]

Medullary: Pertaining to the marrow or to any medulla; resembling marrow. [EU]

Mitoguazone: Antineoplastic agent effective against myelogenous leukemia in experimental animals. Also acts as an inhibitor of animal S-adenosylmethionine decarboxylase. [NIH]

Oncology: The study of cancer. [NIH]

Papillary: Pertaining to or resembling papilla, or nipple. [EU]

Potassium: A metallic element that is important in body functions such as regulation of blood pressure and of water content in cells, transmission of nerve impulses, digestion, muscle contraction, and heart beat. [NIH]

Radioactive: Giving off radiation. [NIH]

Refractory: Not readily yielding to treatment. [EU]

Staging: Performing exams and tests to learn the extent of the cancer within the body, especially whether the disease has spread from the original site to other parts of the body. [NIH]

Systemic: Affecting the entire body. [NIH]

Thyroid: A gland located near the windpipe (trachea) that produces thyroid hormone, which helps regulate growth and metabolism. [NIH]

Tracheostomy: Surgery to create an opening (stoma) into the windpipe. The opening itself may also be called a tracheostomy. [NIH]

CHAPTER 2. SEEKING GUIDANCE

Overview

Some patients are comforted by the knowledge that a number of organizations dedicate their resources to helping people with thyroid cancer. These associations can become invaluable sources of information and advice. Many associations offer aftercare support, financial assistance, and other important services. Furthermore, healthcare research has shown that support groups often help people to better cope with their conditions.[8] In addition to support groups, your physician can be a valuable source of guidance and support. Therefore, finding a physician that can work with your unique situation is a very important aspect of your care.

In this chapter, we direct you to resources that can help you find patient organizations and medical specialists. We begin by describing how to find associations and peer groups that can help you better understand and cope with thyroid cancer. The chapter ends with a discussion on how to find a doctor that is right for you.

Associations and Thyroid Cancer

As mentioned by the Agency for Healthcare Research and Quality, sometimes the emotional side of an illness can be as taxing as the physical side.[9] You may have fears or feel overwhelmed by your situation. Everyone has different ways of dealing with disease or physical injury. Your attitude, your expectations, and how well you cope with your condition can all

---

[8] Churches, synagogues, and other houses of worship might also have groups that can offer you the social support you need.
[9] This section has been adapted from **http://www.ahcpr.gov/consumer/diaginf5.htm**.

influence your well-being. This is true for both minor conditions and serious illnesses. For example, a study on female breast cancer survivors revealed that women who participated in support groups lived longer and experienced better quality of life when compared with women who did not participate. In the support group, women learned coping skills and had the opportunity to share their feelings with other women in the same situation.

There are a number of directories that list additional medical associations that you may find useful. While not all of these directories will provide different information, by consulting all of them, you will have nearly exhausted all sources for patient associations.

The National Cancer Institute (NCI)

The National Cancer Institute (NCI) has complied a list of national organizations that offer services to people with cancer and their families. To view the list, see the NCI fact sheet online at the following Web address: **http://cis.nci.nih.gov/fact/8_1.htm**. The name of each organization is accompanied by its contact information and a brief explanation of its services.

The National Health Information Center (NHIC)

The National Health Information Center (NHIC) offers a free referral service to help people find organizations that provide information about thyroid cancer. For more information, see the NHIC's Web site at **http://www.health.gov/NHIC/** or contact an information specialist by calling 1-800-336-4797.

DIRLINE

A comprehensive source of information on associations is the DIRLINE database maintained by the National Library of Medicine. The database comprises some 10,000 records of organizations, research centers, and government institutes and associations which primarily focus on health and biomedicine. DIRLINE is available via the Internet at the following Web site: **http://dirline.nlm.nih.gov/**. Simply type in "thyroid cancer" (or a synonym) or the name of a topic, and the site will list information contained in the database on all relevant organizations.

The Combined Health Information Database

Another comprehensive source of information on healthcare associations is the Combined Health Information Database. Using the "Detailed Search" option, you will need to limit your search to "Organizations" and "thyroid cancer". Type the following hyperlink into your Web browser: **http://chid.nih.gov/detail/detail.html**. To find associations, use the drop boxes at the bottom of the search page where "You may refine your search by." For publication date, select "All Years." Then, select your preferred language and the format option "Organization Resource Sheet." By making these selections and typing in "thyroid cancer" (or synonyms) into the "For these words:" box, you will only receive results on organizations dealing with thyroid cancer. You should check back periodically with this database since it is updated every 3 months.

The National Organization for Rare Disorders, Inc.

The National Organization for Rare Disorders, Inc. has prepared a Web site that provides, at no charge, lists of associations organized by specific diseases. You can access this database at the following Web site: **http://www.rarediseases.org/cgi-bin/nord/searchpage**. Select the option called 'Organizational Database (ODB)" and type "thyroid cancer" (or a synonym) in the search box.

Cancer Support Groups[10]

People diagnosed with cancer and their families face many challenges that may leave them feeling overwhelmed, afraid, and alone. It can be difficult to cope with these challenges or to talk to even the most supportive family members and friends. Often, support groups can help people affected by cancer feel less alone and can improve their ability to deal with the uncertainties and challenges that cancer brings. Support groups give people who are affected by similar diseases an opportunity to meet and discuss ways to cope with the illness.

---

[10] This section has been adapted from the NCI: **http://cis.nci.nih.gov/fact/8_8.htm**.

How Can Support Groups Help?

People who have been diagnosed with cancer sometimes find they need assistance coping with the emotional as well as the practical aspects of their disease. In fact, attention to the emotional burden of cancer is sometimes part of a patient's treatment plan. Cancer support groups are designed to provide a confidential atmosphere where cancer patients or cancer survivors can discuss the challenges that accompany the illness with others who may have experienced the same challenges. For example, people gather to discuss the emotional needs created by cancer, to exchange information about their disease—including practical problems such as managing side effects or returning to work after treatment—and to share their feelings. Support groups have helped thousands of people cope with these and similar situations.

Can Family Members and Friends Participate in Support Groups?

Family and friends are affected when cancer touches someone they love, and they may need help in dealing with stresses such as family disruptions, financial worries, and changing roles within relationships. To help meet these needs, some support groups are designed just for family members of people diagnosed with cancer; other groups encourage families and friends to participate along with the cancer patient or cancer survivor.

How Can People Find Support Groups?

Many organizations offer support groups for people diagnosed with cancer and their family members or friends. The NCI fact sheet *National Organizations That Offer Services to People with Cancer and Their Families* lists many cancer-concerned organizations that can provide information about support groups. This fact sheet is available at **http://cis.nci.nih.gov/fact/8_1.htm** on the Internet, or can be ordered from the Cancer Information Service at 1-800-4-CANCER (1-800-422-6237). Some of these organizations provide information on their Web sites about contacting support groups.

Doctors, nurses, or hospital social workers who work with cancer patients may also have information about support groups, such as their location, size, type, and how often they meet. Most hospitals have social services departments that provide information about cancer support programs.

Additionally, many newspapers carry a special health supplement containing information about where to find support groups.

What Types of Support Groups Are Available?

Several kinds of support groups are available to meet the individual needs of people at all stages of cancer treatment, from diagnosis through follow-up care. Some groups are general cancer support groups, while more specialized groups may be for teens or young adults, for family members, or for people affected by a particular disease. Support groups may be led by a professional, such as a psychiatrist, psychologist, or social worker, or by cancer patients or survivors. In addition, support groups can vary in approach, size, and how often they meet. Many groups are free, but some require a fee (people can contact their health insurance company to find out whether their plan will cover the cost). It is important for people to find an atmosphere that is comfortable and meets their individual needs.

Online Support Groups

In addition to support groups, commercial Internet service providers offer forums and chat rooms for people with different illnesses and conditions. WebMD®, for example, offers such a service at their Web site: **http://boards.webmd.com/roundtable**. These online self-help communities can help you connect with a network of people whose concerns are similar to yours. Online support groups are places where people can talk informally. If you read about a novel approach, consult with your doctor or other healthcare providers, as the treatments or discoveries you hear about may not be scientifically proven to be safe and effective.

The Cancer Information Service[11]

The Cancer Information Service (CIS) is a program of the National Cancer Institute (NCI), the Nation's lead agency for cancer research. As a resource for information and education about cancer, the CIS is a leader in helping people become active participants in their own health care by providing the latest information on cancer in understandable language. Through its

---

[11] This section has been adapted from the NCI: **http://cis.nci.nih.gov/fact/2_5.htm**.

network of regional offices, the CIS serves the United States, Puerto Rico, the U.S. Virgin Islands, and the Pacific Islands.

For 25 years, the Cancer Information Service has provided the latest and most accurate cancer information to patients and families, the public, and health professionals by:

- Interacting with people one-on-one through its Information Service,
- Working with organizations through its Partnership Program,
- Participating in research efforts to find the best ways to help people adopt healthier behaviors,
- Providing access to NCI information over the Internet.

How Does the CIS Assist the Public?

Through the CIS toll-free telephone service (1–800–4–CANCER), callers speak with knowledgeable, caring staff who are experienced at explaining medical information in easy-to-understand terms. CIS information specialists answer calls in English and Spanish. They also provide cancer information to deaf and hard of hearing callers through the toll-free TTY number (1–800–332–8615). CIS staff have access to comprehensive, accurate information from the NCI on a range of cancer topics, including the most recent advances in cancer treatment. They take as much time as each caller needs, provide thorough and personalized attention, and keep all calls confidential.

The CIS also provides live, online assistance to users of NCI Web sites through LiveHelp, an instant messaging service that is available from 9:00 a.m. to 7:30 p.m. Eastern time, Monday through Friday. Through LiveHelp, information specialists provide answers to questions about cancer and help in navigating Cancer.gov, the NCI's Web site.

Through the telephone numbers or LiveHelp service, CIS users receive:

- Answers to their questions about cancer, including ways to prevent cancer, symptoms and risks, diagnosis, current treatments, and research studies;
- Written materials from the NCI;
- Referrals to clinical trials and cancer-related services, such as treatment centers, mammography facilities, or other cancer organizations;
- Assistance in quitting smoking from information specialists trained in smoking cessation counseling.

What Kind of Assistance Does the CIS Partnership Program Offer?

Through its Partnership Program, the CIS collaborates with established national, state, and regional organizations to reach minority and medically underserved audiences with cancer information. Partnership Program staff provide assistance to organizations developing programs that focus on breast and cervical cancer, clinical trials, tobacco control, and cancer awareness for special populations. To reach those in need, the CIS:

- Helps bring cancer information to people who do not traditionally seek health information or who may have difficulties doing so because of educational, financial, cultural, or language barriers;

- Provides expertise to organizations to help strengthen their ability to inform people they serve about cancer; and

- Links organizations with similar goals and helps them plan and evaluate programs, develop coalitions, conduct training on cancer-related topics, and use NCI resources.

How Do CIS Research Efforts Assist the Public?

The CIS plays an important role in research by studying the most effective ways to communicate with people about healthy lifestyles; health risks; and options for preventing, diagnosing, and treating cancer. The ability to conduct health communications research is a unique aspect of the CIS. Results from these research studies can be applied to improving the way the CIS communicates about cancer and can help other programs communicate more effectively.

How Do People Reach the Cancer Information Service?

- To speak with a CIS information specialist call 1-800-4-CANCER (1-800-422-6237), 9:00 a.m. to 4:30 p.m. local time, Monday through Friday. Deaf or hard of hearing callers with TTY equipment may call 1-800-332-8615.

- To obtain online assistance visit the NCI's Cancer Information Web site at **http://cancer.gov/cancer_information** and click on the LiveHelp link between 9:00 a.m. and 7:30 p.m. Eastern time, Monday through Friday.

- For information 24 hours a day, 7 days a week call 1-800-4-CANCER and select option 4 to hear recorded information at any time.

- Visit NCI's Web site at **http://cancer.gov** on the Internet.

- Visit the CIS Web site at **http://cancer.gov/cis** on the Internet.

Finding Cancer Resources in Your Community[12]

If you have cancer or are undergoing cancer treatment, there are places in your community to turn to for help. There are many local organizations throughout the country that offer a variety of practical and support services to people with cancer. However, people often don't know about these services or are unable to find them. National cancer organizations can assist you in finding these resources, and there are a number of things you can do for yourself.

Whether you are looking for a support group, counseling, advice, financial assistance, transportation to and from treatment, or information about cancer, most neighborhood organizations, local health care providers, or area hospitals are a good place to start. Often, the hardest part of looking for help is knowing the right questions to ask.

What Kind of Help Can I Get?

Until now, you probably never thought about the many issues and difficulties that arise with a diagnosis of cancer. There are support services to help you deal with almost any type of problem that might occur. The first step in finding the help you need is knowing what types of services are available. The following pages describe some of these services and how to find them.

- **Information on Cancer.** Most national cancer organizations provide a range of information services, including materials on different types of cancer, treatments, and treatment-related issues.

- **Counseling.** While some people are reluctant to seek counseling, studies show that having someone to talk to reduces stress and helps people both mentally and physically. Counseling can also provide emotional support to cancer patients and help them better understand their illness. Different types of counseling include individual, group, family, self-help (sometimes called peer counseling), bereavement, patient-to-patient, and sexuality.

- **Medical Treatment Decisions.** Often, people with cancer need to make complicated medical decisions. Many organizations provide hospital and physician referrals for second opinions and information on clinical trials (research studies with people), which may expand treatment options.

---

[12] Adapted from the NCI: **http://cis.nci.nih.gov/fact/8_9.htm**.

- **Prevention and Early Detection.** While cancer prevention may never be 100 percent effective, many things (such as quitting smoking and eating healthy foods) can greatly reduce a person's risk for developing cancer. Prevention services usually focus on smoking cessation and nutrition. Early detection services, which are designed to detect cancer when a person has no symptoms of disease, can include referrals for screening mammograms, Pap tests, or prostate exams.

- **Home Health Care.** Home health care assists patients who no longer need to stay in a hospital or nursing home, but still require professional medical help. Skilled nursing care, physical therapy, social work services, and nutrition counseling are all available at home.

- **Hospice Care.** Hospice is care focused on the special needs of terminally ill cancer patients. Sometimes called *palliative care*, it centers around providing comfort, controlling physical symptoms, and giving emotional support to patients who can no longer benefit from curative treatment. Hospice programs provide services in various settings, including the patient's home, hospice centers, hospitals, or skilled nursing facilities. Your doctor or social worker can provide a referral for these services.

- **Rehabilitation.** Rehabilitation services help people adjust to the effects of cancer and its treatment. Physical rehabilitation focuses on recovery from the physical effects of surgery or the side effects associated with chemotherapy. Occupational or vocational therapy helps people readjust to everyday routines, get back to work, or find employment.

- **Advocacy.** Advocacy is a general term that refers to promoting or protecting the rights and interests of a certain group, such as cancer patients. Advocacy groups may offer services to assist with legal, ethical, medical, employment, legislative, or insurance issues, among others. For instance, if you feel your insurance company has not handled your claim fairly, you may want to advocate for a review of its decision.

- **Financial.** Having cancer can be a tremendous financial burden to cancer patients and their families. There are programs sponsored by the government and nonprofit organizations to help cancer patients with problems related to medical billing, insurance coverage, and reimbursement issues. There are also sources for financial assistance, and ways to get help collecting entitlements from Medicaid, Medicare, and the Social Security Administration.

- **Housing/Lodging.** Some organizations provide lodging for the family of a patient undergoing treatment, especially if it is a child who is ill and the parents are required to accompany the child to treatment.

- **Children's Services.** A number of organizations provide services for children with cancer, including summer camps, make-a-wish programs, and help for parents seeking child care.

How to Find These Services

Often, the services that people with cancer are looking for are right in their own neighborhood or city. The following is a list of places where you can begin your search for help.

- The hospital, clinic, or medical center where you see your doctor, received your diagnosis, or where you undergo treatment should be able to give you information. Your doctor or nurse may be able to tell you about your specific medical condition, pain management, rehabilitation services, home nursing, or hospice care.

- Most hospitals also have a social work, home care, or discharge planning department. This department may be able to help you find a support group, a nonprofit agency that helps people who have cancer, or the government agencies that oversee Social Security, Medicare, and Medicaid. While you are undergoing treatment, be sure to ask the hospital about transportation, practical assistance, or even temporary child care. Talk to a hospital financial counselor in the business office about developing a monthly payment plan if you need help with hospital expenses.

- The public library is an excellent source of information, as are patient libraries at many cancer centers. A librarian can help you find books and articles through a literature search.

- A local church, synagogue, YMCA or YWCA, or fraternal order may provide financial assistance, or may have volunteers who can help with transportation and home care. Catholic Charities, the United Way, or the American Red Cross may also operate local offices. Some of these organizations may provide home care, and the United Way's information and referral service can refer you to an agency that provides financial help. To find the United Way serving your community, visit their online directory at **http://www.unitedway.org** on the Internet or look in the White Pages of your local telephone book.

- Local or county government agencies may offer low-cost transportation (sometimes called para-transit) to individuals unable to use public transportation. Most states also have an Area Agency on Aging that offers low-cost services to people over 60. Your hospital or community social worker can direct you to government agencies for entitlements, including Social Security, state disability, Medicaid, income maintenance, and food stamps. (Keep in mind that most applications to entitlement programs take some time to process.) The Federal government also runs the Hill-Burton program (1-800-638-0742), which funds certain medical facilities and hospitals to provide cancer patients with free or low-cost care if they are in financial need.

Getting the Most From a Service: What To Ask

No matter what type of help you are looking for, the only way to find resources to fit your needs is to ask the right questions. When you are calling an organization for information, it is important to think about what questions you are going to ask before you call. Many people find it helpful to write out their questions in advance, and to take notes during the call. Another good tip is to ask the name of the person with whom you are speaking in case you have follow-up questions. Below are some of the questions you may want to consider if you are calling or visiting a new agency and want to learn about how they can help:

- How do I apply [for this service]?
- Are there eligibility requirements? What are they?
- Is there an application process? How long will it take? What information will I need to complete the application process? Will I need anything else to get the service?
- Do you have any other suggestions or ideas about where I can find help?

The most important thing to remember is that you will rarely receive help unless you ask for it. In fact, asking can be the hardest part of getting help. Don't be afraid or ashamed to ask for assistance. Cancer is a very difficult disease, but there are people and services that can ease your burdens and help you focus on your treatment and recovery.

Finding Doctors Who Specialize in Cancer Care[13]

One of the most important aspects of your treatment will be the relationship between you and your doctor or specialist. All patients with thyroid cancer must go through the process of selecting a physician. A common way to find a doctor who specializes in cancer care is to ask for a referral from your

---

[13] Adapted from the NCI: **http://cis.nci.nih.gov/fact/7_47.htm**.

primary care physician. Sometimes, you may know a specialist yourself, or through the experience of a family member, coworker, or friend.

The following resources may also be able to provide you with names of doctors who specialize in treating specific diseases or conditions. However, these resources may not have information about the quality of care that the doctors provide.

- Your local hospital or its patient referral service may be able to provide you with a list of specialists who practice at that hospital.

- Your nearest National Cancer Institute (NCI)-designated cancer center can provide information about doctors who practice at that center. The NCI fact sheet *The National Cancer Institute Cancer Centers Program* describes and gives contact information, including Web sites, for NCI-designated cancer treatment centers around the country. Many of the cancer centers' Web sites have searchable directories of physicians who practice at each facility. The NCI's fact sheet is available at **http://cis.nci.nih.gov/fact/1_2.htm** on the Internet, or by calling the Cancer Information Service (CIS) at 1-800-4-CANCER (1-800-422-6237).

- The American Board of Medical Specialties (ABMS) publishes a list of board-certified physicians. The *Official ABMS Directory of Board Certified Medical Specialists* lists doctors' names along with their specialty and their educational background. This resource is available in most public libraries. The ABMS also has a Web site that can be used to verify whether a specific physician is board-certified. This free service is located at **http://www.abms.org/newsearch.asp** on the Internet. Verification of a physician's board certification can also be obtained by calling the ABMS at 1-866-275-2267 (1-866-ASK-ABMS).

- The American Medical Association (AMA) provides an online service called AMA Physician Select that offers basic professional information on virtually every licensed physician in the United States and its possessions. The database can be searched by doctor's name or by medical specialty. The AMA Physician Select service is located at **http://www.ama-assn.org/aps/amahg.htm** on the Internet.

- The American Society of Clinical Oncologists (ASCO) provides an online list of doctors who are members of ASCO. The member database has the names and affiliations of over 15,000 oncologists worldwide. It can be searched by doctor's name, institution's name, location, and/or type of board certification. This service is located at **http://www.asco.org/people/db/html/m_db.htm** on the Internet.

- The American College of Surgeons (ACOS) Fellowship Database is an online list of surgeons who are Fellows of the ACOS. The list can be searched by doctor's name, geographic location, or medical specialty. This service is located at **http://web.facs.org/acsdir/default.htm** on the Internet. The ACOS can be contacted at 633 North Saint Clair Street, Chicago, IL 60611-3211; or by telephone at 312-202-5000.
- Local medical societies may maintain lists of doctors in each specialty.
- Public and medical libraries may have print directories of doctors' names, listed geographically by specialty.
- Your local Yellow Pages may have doctors listed by specialty under "Physicians."

The Agency for Healthcare Research and Quality (AHRQ) offers *Your Guide to Choosing Quality Health Care*, which has information for consumers on choosing a health plan, a doctor, a hospital, or a long-term care provider. The Guide includes suggestions and checklists that you can use to determine which doctor or hospital is best for you. This resource is available at **http://www.ahrq.gov/consumer/qntool.htm** on the Internet. You can also order the Guide by calling the AHRQ Publications Clearinghouse at 1-800-358-9295.

If you are a member of a health insurance plan, your choice may be limited to doctors who participate in your plan. Your insurance company can provide you with a list of participating primary care doctors and specialists. It is important to ask your insurance company if the doctor you choose is accepting new patients through your health plan. You also have the option of seeing a doctor outside your health plan and paying the costs yourself. If you have a choice of health insurance plans, you may first wish to consider which doctor or doctors you would like to use, then choose a plan that includes your chosen physician(s).

The National Comprehensive Cancer Network (NCCN) Physician Directory lists specialists who practice in the NCCN's 19 member institutions across the U.S. To access the directory, go to **http://www.nccn.org/** and click on "Physician Directory". To use this service, you will be required to scroll to the bottom of the page and select "I agree." Enter your search criteria and select "Find" at the bottom of the page. To obtain more information on a physician or institution, contact the institution's Physician Referral Department or the NCCN Patient Information and Referral Service at 1-888-909-NCCN or **patientinformation@nccn.org**.

If the previous sources did not meet your needs, you may want to log on to the Web site of the National Organization for Rare Disorders (NORD) at **http://www.rarediseases.org/**. NORD maintains a database of doctors with expertise in various rare diseases. The Metabolic Information Network (MIN), 800-945-2188, also maintains a database of physicians with expertise in various metabolic diseases.

Selecting Your Doctor[14]

There are many factors to consider when choosing a doctor. To make the most informed decision, you may wish to speak with several doctors before choosing one. When you meet with each doctor, you might want to consider the following:

- Does the doctor have the education and training to meet my needs?
- Does the doctor use the hospital that I have chosen?
- Does the doctor listen to me and treat me with respect?
- Does the doctor explain things clearly and encourage me to ask questions?
- What are the doctor's office hours?
- Who covers for the doctor when he or she is unavailable? Will that person have access to my medical records?
- How long does it take to get an appointment with the doctor?

If you are choosing a surgeon, you may wish to ask additional questions about the surgeon's background and experience with specific procedures. These questions may include:

- Is the surgeon board-certified?[15]
- Has the surgeon been evaluated by a national professional association of surgeons, such as the American College of Surgeons (ACOS)?
- At which treatment facility or facilities does the surgeon practice?
- How often does the surgeon perform the type of surgery I need?

---

[14] This section has been adapted from the AHRQ: http://www.ahrq.gov/consumer/qntascii/qntdr.htm
[15] While board certification is a good measure of a doctor's knowledge, it is possible to receive quality care from doctors who are not board certified.

- How many of these procedures has the surgeon performed? What was the success rate?

It is important for you to feel comfortable with the specialist that you choose, because you will be working closely with that person to make decisions about your cancer treatment. Trust your own observations and feelings when deciding on a doctor for your medical care.

Other health professionals and support services may also be important during cancer treatment. The National Cancer Institute fact sheet *Your Health Care Team: Your Doctor Is Only the Beginning* has information about these providers and services, and how to locate them. This fact sheet is located at **http://cis.nci.nih.gov/fact/8_10.htm** on the Internet, or can be obtained by calling the CIS at 1-800-4-CANCER (1-800-422-6237).

Working with Your Doctor[16]

Research has shown that patients who have good relationships with their doctors tend to be more satisfied with their care and have better results. Here are some tips to help you and your doctor become partners:

- You know important things about your symptoms and your health history. Tell your doctor what you think he or she needs to know.
- It is important to tell your doctor personal information, even if it makes you feel embarrassed or uncomfortable.
- Bring a "health history" list with you (and keep it up to date).
- Always bring any medications you are currently taking with you to the appointment, or you can bring a list of your medications including dosage and frequency information. Talk about any allergies or reactions you have had to your medications.
- Tell your doctor about any natural or alternative medicines you are taking.
- Bring other medical information, such as x-ray films, test results, and medical records.
- Ask questions. If you don't, your doctor will assume that you understood everything that was said.

---

[16] This section has been adapted from the AHRQ:
www.ahrq.gov/consumer/qntascii/qntdr.htm.

- Write down your questions before your visit. List the most important ones first to make sure that they are addressed.

- Consider bringing a friend with you to the appointment to help you ask questions. This person can also help you understand and/or remember the answers.

- Ask your doctor to draw pictures if you think that this would help you understand.

- Take notes. Some doctors do not mind if you bring a tape recorder to help you remember things, but always ask first.

- Let your doctor know if you need more time. If there is not time that day, perhaps you can speak to a nurse or physician assistant on staff or schedule a telephone appointment.

- Take information home. Ask for written instructions. Your doctor may also have brochures and audio and videotapes that can help you.

- After leaving the doctor's office, take responsibility for your care. If you have questions, call. If your symptoms get worse or if you have problems with your medication, call. If you had tests and do not hear from your doctor, call for your test results. If your doctor recommended that you have certain tests, schedule an appointment to get them done. If your doctor said you should see an additional specialist, make an appointment.

By following these steps, you will enhance the relationship you will have with your physician.

Finding a Cancer Treatment Facility[17]

Choosing a treatment facility is another important consideration for getting the best medical care possible. Although you may not be able to choose which hospital treats you in an emergency, you can choose a facility for scheduled and ongoing care. If you have already found a doctor for your cancer treatment, you may need to choose a facility based on where your doctor practices. Your doctor may be able to recommend a facility that provides quality care to meet your needs. You may wish to ask the following questions when considering a treatment facility:

- Has the facility had experience and success in treating my condition?

---

[17] Adapted from the NCI: **http://cis.nci.nih.gov/fact/7_47.htm**. At this Web site, information on how to find treatment facilities is also available for patients living outside the U.S.

- Has the facility been rated by state, consumer, or other groups for its quality of care?
- How does the facility check and work to improve its quality of care?
- Has the facility been approved by a nationally recognized accrediting body, such as the American College of Surgeons (ACOS) and/or the Joint Commission on Accredited Healthcare Organizations (JCAHO)?
- Does the facility explain patients' rights and responsibilities? Are copies of this information available to patients?
- Does the treatment facility offer support services, such as social workers and resources to help me find financial assistance if I need it?
- Is the facility conveniently located?

If you are a member of a health insurance plan, your choice of treatment facilities may be limited to those that participate in your plan. Your insurance company can provide you with a list of approved facilities. Although the costs of cancer treatment can be very high, you have the option of paying out-of-pocket if you want to use a treatment facility that is not covered by your insurance plan. If you are considering paying for treatment yourself, you may wish to discuss the potential costs with your doctor beforehand. You may also want to speak with the person who does the billing for the treatment facility. In some instances, nurses and social workers can provide you with more information about coverage, eligibility, and insurance issues.

The following resources may help you find a hospital or treatment facility for your care:

- The NCI fact sheet *The National Cancer Institute Cancer Centers Program* describes and gives contact information for NCI-designated cancer treatment centers around the country.
- The ACOS accredits cancer programs at hospitals and other treatment facilities. More than 1,400 programs in the United States have been designated by the ACOS as Approved Cancer Programs. The ACOS Web site offers a searchable database of these programs at **http://web.facs.org/cpm/default.htm** on the Internet. The ACOS can be contacted at 633 North Saint Clair Street, Chicago, IL 60611-3211; or by telephone at 312-202-5000.
- The JCAHO is an independent, not-for-profit organization that evaluates and accredits health care organizations and programs in the United States. It also offers information for the general public about choosing a

treatment facility. The JCAHO Web site is located at **http://www.jcaho.org** on the Internet. The JCAHO is located at One Renaissance Boulevard, Oakbrook Terrace, IL 60181-4294. The telephone number is 630-792-5800.

- The JCAHO offers an online Quality Check service that patients can use to determine whether a specific facility has been accredited by the JCAHO and view the organization's performance reports. This service is located at **http://www.jcaho.org/qualitycheck/directry/directry.asp** on the Internet.

- The AHRQ publication *Your Guide To Choosing Quality Health Care* has suggestions and checklists for choosing the treatment facility that is right for you.

Additional Cancer Support Information

In addition to the references above, the NCI has set up guidance Web sites that offers information on issues relating to cancer. These include:

- Facing Forward - A Guide for Cancer Survivors:
  http://www.cancer.gov/cancer_information/doc_img.aspx?viewid=cc93a843-6fc0-409e-8798-5c65afc172fe

- Taking Time: Support for People With Cancer and the People Who Care About Them:
  http://www.cancer.gov/cancer_information/doc_img.aspx?viewid=21a46445-a5c8-4fee-95a3-d9d0d665077a

- When Cancer Recurs: Meeting the Challenge:
  http://www.cancer.gov/cancer_information/doc_img.aspx?viewid=9e13d0d2-b7de-4bd6-87da-5750300a0dab

- Your Health Care Team: Your Doctor Is Only the Beginning:
  http://cis.nci.nih.gov/fact/8_10.htm

Vocabulary Builder

The following vocabulary builder provides definitions of words used in this chapter that have not been defined in previous chapters:

Bereavement: Refers to the whole process of grieving and mourning and is associated with a deep sense of loss and sadness. [NIH]

Cervical: Relating to the neck, or to the neck of any organ or structure.

Cervical lymph nodes are located in the neck; cervical cancer refers to cancer of the uterine cervix, which is the lower, narrow end (the "neck") of the uterus. [NIH]

Charities: Social welfare organizations with programs designed to assist individuals in times of need. [NIH]

Curative: Tending to overcome disease and promote recovery. [EU]

Mammogram: An x-ray of the breast. [NIH]

Mammography: The use of x-rays to create a picture of the breast. [NIH]

Oncologist: A doctor who specializes in treating cancer. Some oncologists specialize in a particular type of cancer treatment. For example, a radiation oncologist specializes in treating cancer with radiation. [NIH]

Palliative: 1. affording relief, but not cure. 2. an alleviating medicine. [EU]

Pap test: The collection of cells from the cervix for examination under a microscope. It is used to detect changes that may be cancer or may lead to cancer, and can show noncancerous conditions, such as infection or inflammation. Also called a Pap smear. [NIH]

Prostate: A gland in males that surrounds the neck of the bladder and the urethra. It secretes a substance that liquifies coagulated semen. It is situated in the pelvic cavity behind the lower part of the pubic symphysis, above the deep layer of the triangular ligament, and rests upon the rectum. [NIH]

Screening: Checking for disease when there are no symptoms. [NIH]

CHAPTER 3. CLINICAL TRIALS AND THYROID CANCER

Overview

Very few medical conditions have a single treatment. The basic treatment guidelines that your physician has discussed with you, or those that you have found using the techniques discussed in Chapter 1, may provide you with all that you will require. For some patients, current treatments can be enhanced with new or innovative techniques currently under investigation. In this chapter, we will describe how clinical trials work and show you how to keep informed of trials concerning thyroid cancer.

What Is a Clinical Trial?[18]

Clinical trials involve the participation of people in medical research. Most medical research begins with studies in test tubes and on animals. Treatments that show promise in these early studies may then be tried with people. The only sure way to find out whether a new treatment is safe, effective, and better than other treatments for thyroid cancer is to try it on patients in a clinical trial.

---

[18] The discussion in this chapter has been adapted from the NIH and the NEI: www.nei.nih.gov/netrials/ctivr.htm.

What Kinds of Clinical Trials Are There?

Clinical trials are carried out in three phases:

- **Phase I.** Researchers first conduct Phase I trials with small numbers of patients and healthy volunteers. If the new treatment is a medication, researchers also try to determine how much of it can be given safely.

- **Phase II.** Researchers conduct Phase II trials in small numbers of patients to find out the effect of a new treatment on thyroid cancer.

- **Phase III.** Finally, researchers conduct Phase III trials to find out how new treatments for thyroid cancer compare with standard treatments already being used. Phase III trials also help to determine if new treatments have any side effects. These trials--which may involve hundreds, perhaps thousands, of people--can also compare new treatments with no treatment.

How Is a Clinical Trial Conducted?

Various organizations support clinical trials at medical centers, hospitals, universities, and doctors' offices across the United States. The "principal investigator" is the researcher in charge of the study at each facility participating in the clinical trial. Most clinical trial researchers are medical doctors, academic researchers, and specialists. The "clinic coordinator" knows all about how the study works and makes all the arrangements for your visits.

All doctors and researchers who take part in the study on thyroid cancer carefully follow a detailed treatment plan called a protocol. This plan fully explains how the doctors will treat you in the study. The "protocol" ensures that all patients are treated in the same way, no matter where they receive care.

Clinical trials are controlled. This means that researchers compare the effects of the new treatment with those of the standard treatment. In some cases, when no standard treatment exists, the new treatment is compared with no treatment. Patients who receive the new treatment are in the treatment group. Patients who receive a standard treatment or no treatment are in the "control" group. In some clinical trials, patients in the treatment group get a new medication while those in the control group get a placebo. A placebo is a harmless substance, a "dummy" pill, that has no effect on thyroid cancer. In other clinical trials, where a new surgery or device (not a medicine) is being tested, patients in the control group may receive a "sham treatment."

This treatment, like a placebo, has no effect on thyroid cancer and does not harm patients.

Researchers assign patients "randomly" to the treatment or control group. This is like flipping a coin to decide which patients are in each group. If you choose to participate in a clinical trial, you will not know which group you will be appointed to. The chance of any patient getting the new treatment is about 50 percent. You cannot request to receive the new treatment instead of the placebo or sham treatment. Often, you will not know until the study is over whether you have been in the treatment group or the control group. This is called a "masked" study. In some trials, neither doctors nor patients know who is getting which treatment. This is called a "double masked" study. These types of trials help to ensure that the perceptions of the patients or doctors will not affect the study results.

Natural History Studies

Unlike clinical trials in which patient volunteers may receive new treatments, natural history studies provide important information to researchers on how thyroid cancer develops over time. A natural history study follows patient volunteers to see how factors such as age, sex, race, or family history might make some people more or less at risk for thyroid cancer. A natural history study may also tell researchers if diet, lifestyle, or occupation affects how a disease or disorder develops and progresses. Results from these studies provide information that helps answer questions such as: How fast will a disease or disorder usually progress? How bad will the condition become? Will treatment be needed?

What Is Expected of Patients in a Clinical Trial?

Not everyone can take part in a clinical trial for a specific disease or disorder. Each study enrolls patients with certain features or eligibility criteria. These criteria may include the type and stage of disease or disorder, as well as, the age and previous treatment history of the patient. You or your doctor can contact the sponsoring organization to find out more about specific clinical trials and their eligibility criteria. If you are interested in joining a clinical trial, your doctor must contact one of the trial's investigators and provide details about your diagnosis and medical history.

If you participate in a clinical trial, you may be required to have a number of medical tests. You may also need to take medications and/or undergo surgery. Depending upon the treatment and the examination procedure, you may be required to receive inpatient hospital care. Or, you may have to return to the medical facility for follow-up examinations. These exams help find out how well the treatment is working. Follow-up studies can take months or years. However, the success of the clinical trial often depends on learning what happens to patients over a long period of time. Only patients who continue to return for follow-up examinations can provide this important long-term information.

Recent Trials on Thyroid Cancer

The National Institutes of Health and other organizations sponsor trials on various diseases and disorders. Because funding for research goes to the medical areas that show promising research opportunities, it is not possible for the NIH or others to sponsor clinical trials for every disease and disorder at all times. The following lists recent trials dedicated to thyroid cancer.[19] If the trial listed by the NIH is still recruiting, you may be eligible. If it is no longer recruiting or has been completed, then you can contact the sponsors to learn more about the study and, if published, the results. Further information on the trial is available at the Web site indicated. Please note that some trials may no longer be recruiting patients or are otherwise closed. Before contacting sponsors of a clinical trial, consult with your physician who can help you determine if you might benefit from participation.

- **Chlorambucil Compared With Radiation Therapy in Treating Patients With Previously Untreated Stage III or Stage IV Follicular Lymphoma**

    Condition(s): stage III grade II follicular mixed cell lymphoma; stage IV grade II follicular mixed cell lymphoma; stage III grade I follicular small cleaved cell lymphoma; stage IV grade III follicular large cell lymphoma; stage IV grade I follicular small cleaved cell lymphoma; stage III grade III follicular large cell lymphoma

    Study Status: This study is currently recruiting patients.

    Sponsor(s): Stichting Hemato-Oncologie voor Volwassenen Nederland

    Purpose - Excerpt: Rationale: Drugs used in chemotherapy use different ways to stop cancer cells from dividing so they stop growing or die. Radiation therapy uses high-energy x-rays to damage cancer cells. It is not yet known if chlorambucil is more effective than radiation therapy in treating follicular lymphoma. Purpose: Randomized phase III trial to compare the effectiveness of chlorambucil with that of radiation therapy

---

[19] These are listed at **www.ClinicalTrials.gov**.

in treating patients who have stage III or stage IV follicular lymphoma that has not been previously treated.

Phase(s): Phase III

Study Type: Treatment

Contact(s): see Web site below

Web Site: http://clinicaltrials.gov/ct/gui/show/NCT00028691;jsessionid=3E1F884EF6F44B6D8BAEA209A74BFD04

Benefits and Risks[20]

What Are the Benefits of Participating in a Clinical Trial?

If you are interested in a clinical trial, it is important to realize that your participation can bring many benefits to you and society at large:

- A new treatment could be more effective than the current treatment for thyroid cancer. Although only half of the participants in a clinical trial receive the experimental treatment, if the new treatment is proved to be more effective and safer than the current treatment, then those patients who did not receive the new treatment during the dinical trial may be among the first to benefit from it when the study is over.

- If the treatment is effective, then it may improve health or prevent diseases or disorders.

- Clinical trial patients receive the highest quality of medical care. Experts watch them closely during the study and may continue to follow them after the study is over.

- People who take part in trials contribute to scientific discoveries that may help other people with thyroid cancer. In cases where certain diseases or disorders run in families, your participation may lead to better care or prevention for your family members.

---

[20] This section has been adapted from ClinicalTrials.gov, a service of the National Institutes of Health:
http://www.clinicaltrials.gov/ct/gui/c/a1r/info/whatis?JServSessionIdzone_ct=9jmun6f291.

The Informed Consent

Once you agree to take part in a clinical trial, you will be asked to sign an "informed consent." This document explains a clinical trial's risks and benefits, the researcher's expectations of you, and your rights as a patient.

What Are the Risks?

Clinical trials may involve risks as well as benefits. Whether or not a new treatment will work cannot be known ahead of time. There is always a chance that a new treatment may not work better than a standard treatment. There is also the possibility that it may be harmful. The treatment you receive may cause side effects that are serious enough to require medical attention.

How Is Patient Safety Protected?

Clinical trials can raise fears of the unknown. Understanding the safeguards that protect patients can ease some of these fears. Before a clinical trial begins, researchers must get approval from their hospital's Institutional Review Board (IRB), an advisory group that makes sure a clinical trial is designed to protect patient safety. During a clinical trial, doctors will closely watch you to see if the treatment is working and if you are experiencing any side effects. All the results are carefully recorded and reviewed. In many cases, experts from the Data and Safety Monitoring Committee carefully monitor each clinical trial and can recommend that a study be stopped at any time. You will only be asked to take part in a dinical trial as a volunteer giving informed consent.

What Are a Patient's Rights in a Clinical Trial?

If you are eligible for a clinical trial, you will be given information to help you decide whether or not you want to participate. As a patient, you have the right to:

- Information on all known risks and benefits of the treatments in the study.
- Know how the researchers plan to carry out the study, for how long, and where.
- Know what is expected of you.

- Know any costs involved for you or your insurance provider.
- Know before any of your medical or personal information is shared with other researchers involved in the clinical trial.
- Talk openly with doctors and ask any questions.

After you join a clinical trial, you have the right to:

- Leave the study at any time. Participation is strictly voluntary. However, you should not enroll if you do not plan to complete the study.
- Receive any new information about the new treatment.
- Continue to ask questions and get answers.
- Maintain your privacy. Your name will not appear in any reports based on the study.
- Know whether you participated in the treatment group or the control group (once the study has been completed).

What Should You Ask before Deciding to Join a Clinical Trial?

Questions you should ask when thinking about joining a clinical trial include the following:

- What is the purpose of the clinical trial?
- What are the standard treatments for thyroid cancer? Why do researchers think the new treatment may be better? What is likely to happen to me with or without the new treatment?
- What tests and treatments will I need? Will I need surgery? Medication? Hospitalization?
- How long will the treatment last? How often will I have to come back for follow-up exams?
- What are the treatment's possible benefits to my condition? What are the short- and long-term risks? What are the possible side effects?
- Will the treatment be uncomfortable? Will it make me feel sick? If so, for how long?
- How will my health be monitored?
- Where will I need to go for the clinical trial? How will I get there?
- How much will it cost to be in the study? What costs are covered by the study? How much will my health insurance cover?

- Will I be able to see my own doctor? Who will be in charge of my care?
- Will taking part in the study affect my daily life? Do I have time to participate?
- How do I feel about taking part in a clinical trial? Are there family members or friends who may benefit from my contributions to new medical knowledge?

Clinical Trials and Insurance Coverage[21]

As you consider enrolling in a clinical trial, you will face the critical issue of how to cover the costs of care. Even if you have health insurance, your coverage may not include some or all of the patient care costs associated with a clinical trial. This is because some health plans define clinical trials as "experimental" or "investigational" procedures.

Because lack of coverage for these costs can keep people from enrolling in trials, the National Cancer Institute is working with major health plans and managed care groups to find solutions. In the meantime, there are strategies that may help you deal with cost and coverage barriers. This section answers frequently asked questions about insurance coverage for clinical trial participation and directs you to additional information resources.

The material here is mainly concerned with treatment clinical trials, since other types of trials (prevention, screening, etc.) are newer and generally not covered by health insurance at all. However, this guide may become more relevant for prevention and other types of trials as these trials grow more common.

If you do not have any health insurance, you may find this section helpful for understanding some of the costs that trials involve.

What Costs Do Trials Involve? Who Is Usually Responsible for Paying Them?

There are two types of costs associated with a trial: patient care costs and research costs.
Patient care costs fall into two categories:

---
[21] Adapted from the NCI:
http://www.cancer.gov/clinical_trials/doc_header.aspx?viewid=1d92be79-8748-4bda-8005-2a56d332463b.

- Usual care costs, such as doctor visits, hospital stays, clinical laboratory tests, x-rays, etc., which occur whether you are participating in a trial or receiving standard treatment. These costs have usually been covered by a third-party health plan, such as Medicare or private insurance.
- Extra care costs associated with clinical trial participation, such as the additional tests that may or may not be fully covered by the clinical trial sponsor and/or research institution.

The sponsor and the participant's health plan need to resolve coverage of these costs for particular trials.

Research costs are those associated with conducting the trial, such as data collection and management, research physician and nurse time, analysis of results, and tests purely performed for research purposes. Such costs are usually covered by the sponsoring organization, such as NCI or a pharmaceutical company.

Criteria Used by Health Plans to Make Reimbursement Decisions about Trials

Health insurance companies and managed care companies decide which health care services they will pay for by developing coverage policy regarding the specific services. In general, the most important factor determining whether something is covered is a health plan's judgment as to whether the service is established or investigational. Health plans usually designate a service as established if there is a certain amount of scientific data to show that it is safe and effective. If the health plan does not think that such data exist in sufficient quantity, the plan may label the service as investigational.

Health care services delivered within the setting of a clinical trial are very often categorized as investigational and not covered. This is because the health plan thinks that the major reason to perform the clinical trial is that there is not enough data to establish the safety and effectiveness of the service being studied. Thus, for some health plans, any mention of the fact that the patient is involved in a clinical trial results in a denial of payment.

Your health plan may define specific criteria that a trial must meet before extending coverage, such as the following:

Sponsorship

Some plans may only cover costs of trials sponsored by organizations whose review and oversight of the trial is careful and scientifically rigorous, according to standards set by the health plan.

Trial Phase and Type

Some plans may cover patient care costs only for the clinical trials they judge to be "medically necessary" on a case-by-case basis. Trial phase may also affect coverage; for example, while a plan may be willing to cover costs associated with Phase III trials, which include treatments that have already been successful with a certain number of people, the plan may require some documentation of effectiveness before covering a Phase I or II trial.

While health plans are interested in efforts to improve prevention and screening, they currently seem less likely to have a review process in place for these trials. Therefore, it may be more difficult to get coverage for the care costs associated with them.

Some plans, especially smaller ones, will not cover any costs associated with a clinical trial. Policies vary widely, but in most cases your best bet is to have your doctor initiate discussions with the health plan.

Cost "Neutrality"

Some health plans may limit coverage to trials they consider cost-neutral (i.e., not significantly more expensive than the treatments considered standard).

Lack of Standard Therapy

Some plans limit coverage of trials to situations in which no standard therapy is available.

Facility and Personnel Qualifications

A health plan may require that the facility and medical staff meet specific qualifications to conduct a trial involving unique services, especially intensive therapy such as a bone marrow transplant (high-dose chemotherapy with bone marrow/ stem cell rescue).

Clinical Trials and Medicare Coverage

For up-to-date information about Medicare coverage of clinical trials, go to the Web site for the Centers for Medicaid & Medicare (**http://www.hcfa.gov/coverage/8d.htm**; formerly the Health Care Financing Administration). As of January 2001, the following information was accurate[22]:

What Will Medicare Pay?

- Anything normally covered is still covered when it is part of a clinical trial. This includes test, procedures, and doctor visits that are ordinarily covered.

- Anything normally covered even if it is a service or item associated with the experimental treatment. For example, Medicare will pay for the intravenous administration of a new chemotherapy drug being tested in a trial, including any therapy to prevent side effects from the new drug.

- Anything normally covered even if it resulted from your being in the clinical trial. For example, a test or hospitalization resulting from a side effect of the new treatment that Medicare would ordinarily cover.

What Costs Are Not Covered?

- Investigational items or services being tested in a trial. Sponsors of clinical trials often provide the new drug free, but make sure you ask your doctor before you begin.

- Items or services used solely for the data collection needs of the trial.

- Anything being provided free by the sponsor of the trial.

---

[22] On June 7, 2000, Present Clinton announced that Medicare would revise its payment policy to reimburse the routine patient care costs of clinical trials. The announcement is available for public viewing at the following Web address:
http://www.cancer.gov/clinical_trials/doc.aspx?viewid=320DD013-BA7A-4177-A000-2011089F34A0.

What Kinds of Clinical Trials Are Covered?

NCI's Cancer Information Service has provided a fact sheet for Medicare beneficiaries at the following Web site: **http://cis.nci.nih.gov/fact/8_14.htm**. In general, cancer treatment and diagnosis trials are covered if:

- They are funded by the National Cancer Institute (NCI), NCI-Designated Cancer Centers, NCI-Sponsored Clinical Trials Cooperative Groups and all other Federal agencies that fund cancer research. Other trials may be eligible for coverage and doctors can ask Medicare to pay the patients' costs. Ask your doctor about this before you begin.

- They are designed to treat or diagnose your cancer.

- The purpose or subject of the trial is within a Medicare benefit category. For example, cancer diagnosis and treatment are Medicare benefits, so these trials are covered. Cancer prevention trials are not currently covered.

Increasing the Likelihood of Insurance Coverage for Trials[23]

There are several steps you can follow to deal with coverage issues up front when deciding to enter a clinical trial. Along the way, enlist the help of family members and your doctor or other health professionals. You may find the following checklist useful:

Understand the Costs Associated with the Trial

Ask your doctor or the trial's contact person about the costs that must be covered by you or your health plan. Are these costs significantly higher than those associated with standard care? Also, inquire about the experience of other patients in the trial. Have their plans paid for their care? Have there been any persistent problems with coverage? How often have the trial's administrators been successful in getting plans to cover patient care costs?

---

[23] This section has been adapted from the NCI:
http://www.cancer.gov/clinical_trials/doc_header.aspx?viewid=1d92be79-8748-4bda-8005-2a56d332463b&docid=0df4397a-eccb-465f-bd33-a89e7a708c46.

Understand Your Health Plan

Be sure you know what's in your policy; request and carefully review the actual contract language. If there's a specific exclusion for "experimental treatment," look closely at the policy to see how the plan defines such treatment and under what conditions it might be covered. If it is not clearly defined, call the plan's customer service line, consult their Web site, and/or write to them. Ask for specific information about clinical trials coverage.

Work Closely with Your Doctor

Talk with your doctor about the paperwork he or she submits to your health plan. If there have been problems with coverage in the past, you might ask your doctor or the hospital to send an information package to the plan that includes studies supporting the procedure's safety, benefits, and medical appropriateness. This package might include:

- Publications from peer-reviewed literature about the proposed therapy that demonstrate patient benefits;
- A letter that uses the insurance contract's own language to explain why the treatment, screening method, or preventive measure should be covered;
- Letters from researchers that explain the clinical trial;
- Support letters from patient advocacy groups.

Be sure to keep your own copy of any materials that the doctor sends to your health plan for future reference.

Work Closely with Your Company's Benefits Manager

This person may be helpful in enlisting the support of your employer to request coverage by the health plan.

Give Your Health Plan a Deadline

Ask the hospital or cancer center to set a target date for the therapy. This will help to ensure that coverage decisions are made promptly.

Know Your Rights[24]

A number of state governments are addressing the question of whether insurance companies ought to cover the costs associated with patients' participation in clinical trials. Lack of such coverage is a significant barrier to many patients who might otherwise benefit from enrolling in a trial. Lack of coverage also makes it harder for researchers to successfully conduct trials that could improve prevention and treatment options. Information on State initiatives and legislation concerning cancer-related clinical trials is available at **http://www.cancer.gov/ClinicalTrials/insurancelaws**. By conducting your own research and learning about your rights, you may increase the likelihood that your insurance company will cover the costs of a trial.

If Your Insurance Claim Is Denied after the Trial Has Begun

If a claim is denied, read your policy to find out what steps you can follow to make an appeal. In "What Cancer Survivors Need to Know about Health Insurance", the National Coalition for Cancer Survivorship suggests that you and your doctor demonstrate to the health plan that:

- The therapy is not just a research study, but also a valid procedure that benefits patients;
- Your situation is similar to that of other patients who are participating in clinical trials as part of a covered benefit;
- Possible complications have been anticipated and can be handled effectively.

You also may wish to contact your state insurance counseling hotline or insurance department for more help, or write your state insurance commissioner describing the problem.

Where Else Can I Turn for Assistance?

It's never easy to deal with financial issues when you or a loved one faces cancer. Unfortunately, costs can present a significant barrier to clinical trials participation. The range of insurance issues and health plan contracts makes it impossible to deal with all of them here. You may wish to consult this partial list of publications, organizations, and Web sites for more information:

---

[24] Adapted from Cancer.gov: **http://www.cancer.gov/ClinicalTrials/insurancelaws**.

Publications

What Cancer Survivors Need to Know about Health Insurance
National Coalition of Cancer Survivorship
1010 Wayne Avenue, 5th floor
Silver Spring, MD 20910
(301) 650-8868
http://www.cansearch.org/

Cancer Treatments Your Insurance Should Cover
The Association of Community Cancer Centers
11600 Nebel Street, Suite 201
Rockville, MD 20852
(301) 984-9496
http://www.accc-cancer.org/main2001.shtml

The Managed Care Answer Guide
Patient Advocate Foundation
739 Thimble Shoals Boulevard, Suite 704
Newport News, VA 23606
(757) 873-6668
E-mail: **ndepaf@pinn.net**

1998 Guide to Health Insurance for People with Medicare, The Medicare Handbook
Medicare Helpline: 1-800-444-4606
Health Care Financing Administration: **http://www.hcfa.gov/**
New Medicare site: **http://www.medicare.gov/**

Assistance Programs

Candlelighters Childhood Cancer Foundation
Ombudsman Program
910 Woodmont Avenue, #4607
Bethesda, MD 20814
(301) 657-8401; 1-800-366-2223 (toll-free)
E-mail: **info@candlelighters.org**
http://www.candlelighters.org
The Ombudsman Program helps families of children with cancer and survivors of childhood cancer resolve a range of problems, including insurance coverage difficulties. Local groups appoint a Parent Advocate who works with the treatment center on behalf of families.

Medical Care Management Corporation
5272 River Road, Suite 650
Bethesda, MD 20816-1405
(301) 652-1818
email: mcman@mcman.com
http://www.mcman.com/
Working for a range of clients, including health plans, employers, and patients, MCMC conducts independent, objective reviews of high-technology medical care cases to assist in decision-making. While it does charge for its services, MCMC also offers a volunteer program for those who cannot afford to pay.

More Information Resources

OncoLink
A service of the University of Pennsylvania Cancer Center.
http://www.oncolink.com/
In addition to general cancer information, this web site features a section on financial information for patients. Among the topics: viatical settlements, life insurance, a glossary of financial and medical terms, and news about billing and insurance.

American Association of Health Plans
1129 20th Street, NW, Suite 600
Washington, DC 20036-3421
(202) 778-3200
http://www.aahp.org/
The Web site section "For Consumers" includes a fact sheet on clinical research that describes various health plans' efforts to support research initiatives and collaborate with academic health centers and universities.

Health Insurance Association of America
555 13th Street, NW
Washington, DC 20004
(202) 824-1600

- Home page: **http://www.hiaa.org/**

- Consumer Information: **http://www.hiaa.org/consumer/**

- Insurance Counseling Hotlines by State:
  http://www.hiaa.org/consumer/insurance_counsel.cfm

- State Insurance Departments:
  http://www.hiaa.org/consumer/state_insurance.cfm

Government Initiatives to Expand Insurance Coverage for Trials[25]

The good news is that there has been a recent effort in the U.S. to assure clinical trials coverage, with NCI involved in several new initiatives as described below:

NCI-Department of Defense Agreement

An innovative 1996 agreement between NCI and the Department of Defense (DoD) has given thousands of DoD cancer patients more options for care and greater access to state-of-the-art treatments. Patients who are beneficiaries of TRICARE/CHAMPUS, the DoD's health program, are covered for NCI-sponsored Phase II and Phase III clinical treatment trials. NCI and DoD are refining a system that allows physicians and patients to determine quickly what current trials meet their needs and where they are taking place.

NCI-Department of Veterans Affairs Agreement

A 1997 agreement with the Department of Veterans Affairs provides coverage for eligible veterans of the armed services to participate in NCI-sponsored prevention, diagnosis, and treatment studies nationwide. For additional information, see the VA/DoD Beneficiaries Digest Page at http://www.va.gov/cancer.htm.

Midwest Health Plans Agreement

Some NCI Cooperative Groups have reached agreements with several insurers in Wisconsin and Minnesota to provide more than 200,000 people with coverage. This coverage is allocated for patient care costs if they participate in a cooperative group-sponsored trial.

---

[25] Adapted from the NCI:
http://www.cancer.gov/clinical_trials/doc_header.aspx?viewid=1d92be79-8748-4bda-8005-2a56d332463b&docid=d8092601-daf9-4794-8536-3be2712eb6b9.

Pediatric Cancer Care Network

This network, a cooperative agreement among the Children's Cancer Group, the Pediatric Oncology Group, and the Blue Cross Blue Shield System Association (BCBS) nationwide, will ensure that children of BCBS subscribers receive care at designated centers of cancer care excellence and may promote the enrollment of children in Cooperative Group clinical trials.

Keeping Current on Clinical Trials

Various government agencies maintain databases on trials. The U.S. National Institutes of Health, through the National Library of Medicine, has developed ClinicalTrials.gov to provide patients, family members, and physicians with current information about clinical research across the broadest number of diseases and conditions.

The site was launched in February 2000 and currently contains approximately 5,700 clinical studies in over 59,000 locations worldwide, with most studies being conducted in the United States. ClinicalTrials.gov receives about 2 million hits per month and hosts approximately 5,400 visitors daily. To access this database, simply go to their Web site (**www.clinicaltrials.gov**) and search by "thyroid cancer" (or synonyms).

While ClinicalTrials.gov is the most comprehensive listing of NIH-supported clinical trials available, not all trials are in the database. The database is updated regularly, so clinical trials are continually being added. The following is a list of specialty databases affiliated with the National Institutes of Health that offer additional information on trials:

- For clinical studies at the Warren Grant Magnuson Clinical Center located in Bethesda, Maryland, visit their Web site:
  http://clinicalstudies.info.nih.gov/

- For clinical studies conducted at the Bayview Campus in Baltimore, Maryland, visit their Web site:
  http://www.jhbmc.jhu.edu/studies/index.html

- For cancer trials, visit the National Cancer Institute:
  http://cancertrials.nci.nih.gov/

General References

The following references describe clinical trials and experimental medical research. They have been selected to ensure that they are likely to be available from your local or online bookseller or university medical library. These references are usually written for healthcare professionals, so you may consider consulting with a librarian or bookseller who might recommend a particular reference. The following includes some of the most readily available references (sorted alphabetically by title; hyperlinks provide rankings, information and reviews at Amazon.com):

- **A Guide to Patient Recruitment : Today's Best Practices & Proven Strategies** by Diana L. Anderson; Paperback - 350 pages (2001), CenterWatch, Inc.; ISBN: 1930624115;
  http://www.amazon.com/exec/obidos/ASIN/1930624115/icongroupinterna

- **A Step-By-Step Guide to Clinical Trials** by Marilyn Mulay, R.N., M.S., OCN; Spiral-bound - 143 pages Spiral edition (2001), Jones & Bartlett Pub; ISBN: 0763715697;
  http://www.amazon.com/exec/obidos/ASIN/0763715697/icongroupinterna

- **The CenterWatch Directory of Drugs in Clinical Trials** by CenterWatch; Paperback - 656 pages (2000), CenterWatch, Inc.; ISBN: 0967302935;
  http://www.amazon.com/exec/obidos/ASIN/0967302935/icongroupinterna

- **The Complete Guide to Informed Consent in Clinical Trials** by Terry Hartnett (Editor); Paperback - 164 pages (2000), PharmSource Information Services, Inc.; ISBN: 0970153309;
  http://www.amazon.com/exec/obidos/ASIN/0970153309/icongroupinterna

- **Dictionary for Clinical Trials** by Simon Day; Paperback - 228 pages (1999), John Wiley & Sons; ISBN: 0471985961;
  http://www.amazon.com/exec/obidos/ASIN/0471985961/icongroupinterna

- **Extending Medicare Reimbursement in Clinical Trials** by Institute of Medicine Staff (Editor), et al; Paperback 1st edition (2000), National Academy Press; ISBN: 0309068886;
  http://www.amazon.com/exec/obidos/ASIN/0309068886/icongroupinterna

- **Handbook of Clinical Trials** by Marcus Flather (Editor); Paperback (2001), Remedica Pub Ltd; ISBN: 1901346293;
  http://www.amazon.com/exec/obidos/ASIN/1901346293/icongroupinterna

Vocabulary Builder

The following vocabulary builder gives definitions of words used in this chapter that have not been defined in previous chapters:

Abdomen: The part of the body that contains the pancreas, stomach, intestines, liver, gallbladder, and other organs. [NIH]

Allogeneic: Taken from different individuals of the same species. [NIH]

Antibody: A type of protein made by certain white blood cells in response to a foreign substance (antigen). Each antibody can bind to only a specific antigen. The purpose of this binding is to help destroy the antigen. Antibodies can work in several ways, depending on the nature of the antigen. Some antibodies destroy antigens directly. Others make it easier for white blood cells to destroy the antigen. [NIH]

Antineoplastons: Substances isolated from normal human blood and urine being tested as a type of treatment for some tumors and AIDS. [NIH]

Autologous: Taken from an individual's own tissues, cells, or DNA. [NIH]

Bevacizumab: A monoclonal antibody that may prevent the growth of blood vessels from surrounding tissue to a solid tumor. [NIH]

Bexarotene: An anticancer drug used to decrease the growth of some types of cancer cells. Also called LGD1069. [NIH]

Bleomycin: An anticancer drug that belongs to the family of drugs called antitumor antibiotics. [NIH]

Catheter: A flexible tube used to deliver fluids into or withdraw fluids from the body. [NIH]

Chlorambucil: An anticancer drug that belongs to the family of drugs called alkylating agents. [NIH]

CNS: Central nervous system. The brain and spinal cord. [NIH]

Corticosteroids: Hormones that have antitumor activity in lymphomas and lymphoid leukemias; in addition, corticosteroids (steroids) may be used for hormone replacement and for the management of some of the complications of cancer and its treatment. [NIH]

Cutaneous: Having to do with the skin. [NIH]

Cyclophosphamide: An anticancer drug that belongs to the family of drugs called alkylating agents. [NIH]

Cyclosporine: A drug used to help reduce the risk of rejection of organ and bone marrow transplants by the body. It is also used in clinical trials to make cancer cells more sensitive to anticancer drugs. [NIH]

Depsipeptide: Anticancer drugs obtained from microorganisms. [NIH]

Doxorubicin: An anticancer drug that belongs to the family of drugs called antitumor antibiotics. It is an anthracycline. [NIH]

Etoposide: An anticancer drug that is a podophyllotoxin derivative and belongs to the family of drugs called mitotic inhibitors. [NIH]

Filgrastim: A colony-stimulating factor that stimulates the production of neutrophils (a type of white blood cell). It is a cytokine that belongs to the family of drugs called hematopoietic (blood-forming) agents. Also called granulocyte colony-stimulating factor (G-CSF). [NIH]

FR901228: An anticancer drug that belongs to the family of drugs called depsipeptides. [NIH]

Grade: The grade of a tumor depends on how abnormal the cancer cells look under a microscope and how quickly the tumor is likely to grow and spread. Grading systems are different for each type of cancer. [NIH]

Graft: Healthy skin, bone, or other tissue taken from one part of the body and used to replace diseased or injured tissue removed from another part of the body. [NIH]

Infusion: A method of putting fluids, including drugs, into the bloodstream. Also called intravenous infusion. [NIH]

Interferon: A biological response modifier (a substance that can improve the body's natural response to disease). Interferons interfere with the division of cancer cells and can slow tumor growth. There are several types of interferons, including interferon-alpha, -beta, and -gamma. These substances are normally produced by the body. They are also made in the laboratory for use in treating cancer and other diseases. [NIH]

Intraocular: Within the eye. [EU]

Intravenous: IV. Into a vein. [NIH]

Leukemia: Cancer of blood-forming tissue. [NIH]

Lymphocytic: Referring to lymphocytes, a type of white blood cell. [NIH]

Methoxsalen: A drug used in ultraviolet light therapy. [NIH]

Mitoxantrone: An anticancer drug that belongs to the family of drugs called antitumor antibiotics. [NIH]

Mycosis: Any disease caused by a fungus. [EU]

Neutropenia: An abnormal decrease in the number of neutrophils, a type of white blood cell. [NIH]

Oxaliplatin: An anticancer drug that belongs to the family of drugs called platinum compounds. [NIH]

Paclitaxel: An anticancer drug that belongs to the family of drugs called mitotic inhibitors. [NIH]

Pelvis: The lower part of the abdomen, located between the hip bones. [NIH]

Plasma: The clear, yellowish, fluid part of the blood that carries the blood cells. The proteins that form blood clots are in plasma. [NIH]

Platelets: A type of blood cell that helps prevent bleeding by causing blood clots to form. Also called thrombocytes. [NIH]

Prednisolone: A synthetic corticosteroid used in the treatment of blood cell cancers (leukemias) and lymph system cancers (lymphomas). [NIH]

Radiolabeled: Any compound that has been joined with a radioactive substance. [NIH]

Radiotherapy: The treatment of disease by ionizing radiation. [EU]

Randomized: Describes an experiment or clinical trial in which animal or human subjects are assigned by chance to separate groups that compare different treatments. [NIH]

Regimen: A treatment plan that specifies the dosage, the schedule, and the duration of treatment. [NIH]

Rituximab: A type of monoclonal antibody used in cancer detection or therapy. Monoclonal antibodies are laboratory-produced substances that can locate and bind to cancer cells. [NIH]

Sargramostim: A colony-stimulating factor that stimulates the production of blood cells, especially platelets, during chemotherapy. It is a cytokine that belongs to the family of drugs called hematopoietic (blood-forming) agents. Also called GM-CSF. [NIH]

Steroid: A group name for lipids that contain a hydrogenated cyclopentanoperhydrophenanthrene ring system. Some of the substances included in this group are progesterone, adrenocortical hormones, the gonadal hormones, cardiac aglycones, bile acids, sterols (such as cholesterol), toad poisons, saponins, and some of the carcinogenic hydrocarbons. [EU]

Thalidomide: A drug that belongs to the family of drugs called angiogenesis inhibitors. It prevents the growth of new blood vessels into a solid tumor. [NIH]

Tomography: A series of detailed pictures of areas inside the body; the pictures are created by a computer linked to an x-ray machine. [NIH]

Transplantation: The replacement of an organ with one from another person. [NIH]

Urine: Fluid containing water and waste products. Urine is made by the kidneys, stored in the bladder, and leaves the body through the urethra. [NIH]

Vaccine: A substance or group of substances meant to cause the immune system to respond to a tumor or to microorganisms, such as bacteria or viruses. [NIH]

Vincristine: An anticancer drug that belongs to the family of plant drugs called vinca alkaloids. [NIH]

Vinorelbine: An anticancer drug that belongs to the family of plant drugs called vinca alkaloids. [NIH]

PART II: ADDITIONAL RESOURCES AND ADVANCED MATERIAL

ABOUT PART II

In Part II, we introduce you to additional resources and advanced research on thyroid cancer. All too often, patients who conduct their own research are overwhelmed by the difficulty in finding and organizing information. The purpose of the following chapters is to provide you an organized and structured format to help you find additional information resources on thyroid cancer. In Part II, as in Part I, our objective is not to interpret the latest advances on thyroid cancer or render an opinion. Rather, our goal is to give you access to original research and to increase your awareness of sources you may not have already considered. In this way, you will come across the advanced materials often referred to in pamphlets, books, or other general works. Once again, some of this material is technical in nature, so consultation with a professional familiar with thyroid cancer is suggested.

CHAPTER 4. STUDIES ON THYROID CANCER

Overview

Every year, academic studies are published on thyroid cancer or related conditions. Broadly speaking, there are two types of studies. The first are peer reviewed. Generally, the content of these studies has been reviewed by scientists or physicians. Peer-reviewed studies are typically published in scientific journals and are usually available at medical libraries. The second type of studies is non-peer reviewed. These works include summary articles that do not use or report scientific results. These often appear in the popular press, newsletters, or similar periodicals.

In this chapter, we will show you how to locate peer-reviewed references and studies on thyroid cancer. We will begin by discussing research that has been summarized and is free to view by the public via the Internet. We then show you how to generate a bibliography on thyroid cancer and teach you how to keep current on new studies as they are published or undertaken by the scientific community.

The Combined Health Information Database

The Combined Health Information Database summarizes studies across numerous federal agencies. To limit your investigation to research studies and thyroid cancer, you will need to use the advanced search options. First, go to **http://chid.nih.gov/index.html**. From there, select the "Detailed Search" option (or go directly to that page with the following hyperlink: **http://chid.nih.gov/detail/detail.html**). The trick in extracting studies is found in the drop boxes at the bottom of the search page where "You may refine your search by." Select the dates and language you prefer, and the format option "Journal Article." At the top of the search form, select the number of records you would like to see (we recommend 100) and check the box to display "whole records." We recommend that you type in "thyroid cancer" (or synonyms) into the "For these words:" box. Consider using the option "anywhere in record" to make your search as broad as possible. If you want to limit the search to only a particular field, such as the title of the journal, then select this option in the "Search in these fields" drop box. The following is a sample of what you can expect from this type of search:

- **Rise of Cancer Among the Elderly in Hawaii**

    Source: Hawaii Medical Journal. 53(7):188, 190-193, 200, July 1994.

    Summary: Researchers conducted a study to determine if similarities existed between time trends in cancer incidence among elderly persons in Hawaii and trends observed in the mainland United States and to determine if the trends were also comparable among the various ethnic groups living in Hawaii. Researchers determined average annual incidence rates per 100,000 persons over age 65 by sex and ethnicity for the time periods 1973-1977 and 1983-1986 through the Hawaii Tumor Registry (HTR), a population-based central cancer registry. Researchers identified patients through the medical records and admissions departments of hospitals, pathology laboratories, and clinics throughout Hawaii. They ensured quality and completeness of the data through the reabstraction of a sample of the medical records from each hospital, and by extensive edit and logic checks built into the computer software to evaluate consistency and validity of responses. Researchers obtained ethnic classification through self-report at the time of hospitalization. The Hawaii Tumor Registry assigned the primary site of cancer according to the International Classification of Diseases for Oncology adopted in 1976 by the World Health Organization (WHO). Results showed that the largest percentage of increase in incidence occurred for melanoma with a gain of 209 percent between the 2 time periods. The next highest increase took place for brain cancer followed by thyroid cancer, colon cancer, multiple myeloma, and lung cancer. The incidence of all cancers combined increased 27 percent among men and 26 percent among women between the 2 time periods. Melanoma also had the largest percentage of increase among women over age 65, followed by cancers of the liver, ovary, and brain. The cancers with the highest percent increase among men included melanoma, multiple myeloma, and cancers of the brain, thyroid, colon, lung, and prostate. With the exception of thyroid cancer, the risk for developing these cancers had also increased in other parts of the United States. Comparisons across ethnic groups revealed that melanoma increased mainly among whites, lung cancer increased primarily among Hawaiians and whites, colon cancer increased in all ethnic groups, prostate cancer increased in all ethnic groups but minimally among Chinese men, and breast cancer increased in all ethnic groups except elderly Filipino women. 4 figures, 2 tables, 20 references.

Federally Funded Research on Thyroid Cancer

The U.S. Government supports a variety of research studies relating to thyroid cancer and associated conditions. These studies are tracked by the Office of Extramural Research at the National Institutes of Health.[26] CRISP (Computerized Retrieval of Information on Scientific Projects) is a searchable database of federally funded biomedical research projects conducted at universities, hospitals, and other institutions. Visit the CRISP Web site at **http://commons.cit.nih.gov/crisp3/CRISP.Generate_Ticket**. You can perform targeted searches by various criteria including geography, date, as well as topics related to thyroid cancer and related conditions.

For most of the studies, the agencies reporting into CRISP provide summaries or abstracts. As opposed to clinical trial research using patients, many federally funded studies use animals or simulated models to explore thyroid cancer and related conditions. In some cases, therefore, it may be difficult to understand how some basic or fundamental research could eventually translate into medical practice. The following sample is typical of the type of information found when searching the CRISP database for thyroid cancer:

- **Project Title: Mechanisms of RET/PTC Rearrangements in Thyroid Cancer**

  Principal Investigator & Institution: Nikiforov, Yuri E.; Assistant Professor; Pathology and Lab Medicine; University of Cincinnati 2624 Clifton Ave Cincinnati, Oh 45221

  Timing: Fiscal Year 2001; Project Start 1-JUL-2001; Project End 0-JUN-2006

  Summary: (Scanned from the applicant's abstract) Thyroid cancer is the most common form of solid neoplasms known to be associated with

---

[26] Healthcare projects are funded by the National Institutes of Health (NIH), Substance Abuse and Mental Health Services (SAMHSA), Health Resources and Services Administration (HRSA), Food and Drug Administration (FDA), Centers for Disease Control and Prevention (CDCP), Agency for Healthcare Research and Quality (AHRQ), and Office of Assistant Secretary of Health (OASH).

radiation exposure. However, the mechanisms of radiation-induced carcinogenesis are not well understood. The high prevalence of rearrangements of the RET gene has been recently found in post-Chernobyl papillary thyroid carcinomas and in thyroid tumors from patients exposed to therapeutic external radiation. The positions of breakpoints sites in the RET and ELEI genes identified in post-Chernobyl tumors with RETPTC3 rearrangements suggested that these two genes may be aligned across from each other in the nucleus at the time of DNA breaks (Nikiforov et al., Oncogene, 1999). Consistent with this idea, we found that one pair of RET and H4 genes (contributing to RET/PTCI rearrangement) was juxtaposed in 35 percent of inter-phase nuclei of normal thyroid cells. These data suggest that two potentially recombinogenic chromosomal loci may be contiguous to each other in the nucleus predisposing to generation of rearrangement by adjacent double-strand DNA breaks produced by ionizing radiation or other genotoxic agents. The main goal of the current proposal is to explore the role of nuclear architecture and gene proximity in generation of chromosomal rearrangements after radiation exposure. We propose to use two-color FISH and three-dimensional confocal laser-scanning microscopy to determine the frequency of physical proximity of genes, contributing to the major types of RET/PTC rearrangements, in normal human thyroid follicular cells and in other cell lineages. We will establish whether chromosomal organization with respect to these loci is cell-type specific, age-dependent, or varies with cell cycle stage. Any of these parameters could explain in part the high prevalence of thyroid cancer after irradiation, and the higher susceptibility of children. Then, we will expose cultured cells to different doses of ionizing radiation to test directly the relationship between gene proximity and the frequency of radiation-induced RET/PTC rearrangements in vitro. These studies will extend our understanding of the mechanisms of radiation-induced carcinogenesis in the thyroid gland. In addition, they are likely to have importance for a broad range of chromosomal rearrangements found in cancer.

Website: http://commons.cit.nih.gov/crisp3/CRISP.Generate_Ticket

- **Project Title: Radiation Induced Thyroid Cancer**

Principal Investigator & Institution: Schneider, Arthur B.; Professor of Medicine and Chief; Medicine; University of Illinois at Chicago at Chicago Chicago, Il 60612

Timing: Fiscal Year 2000; Project Start 1-APR-1977; Project End 0-JUN-2003

Summary: The major objective of this research proposal is to study radiation- induced thyroid cancer by coordinated clinical, epidemiological and laboratory investigations. The clinical studies are designed to determine the continuing incidence of radiation-induced thyroid cancer and to evaluate methods of diagnosis and medical and surgical approaches to treatment. This will be accomplished by continuing the longitudinal study of patients who received childhood head and neck irradiation for benign conditions at Michael Reese Hospital. Of the 4,296 patients who were so treated 3,058 (71.2 percent) have been located and 1,025 (33.5 percent) have had surgery for thyroid nodules. Among those who have had surgery, 357 (34.8 percent) have had thyroid cancer. The follow-up of this population will continue with the following aims: (1) to determine the continuing incidence of radiation-induced thyroid cancer, (2) to determine if their radiation-induced thyroid cancers have the same age- dependent worsening prognosis as seen in the general population, and (3) to evaluate the diagnostic methods and treatment methods that have been used. Laboratory studies will focus on the role of serum thyroglobulin in the diagnosis of thyroid tumors. Parallel studies will continue on other radiation-induced tumors, including benign and malignant salivary tumors, neural tumors, parathyroid tumors and others. Together these will provide the information to develop guidelines for the care of persons with a history of radiation. Epidemiological studies will focus on identifying evidence for the existence of heritable radiation susceptibility factors. Patterns of multiple tumors in irradiated individuals and family histories of cancer will be analyzed. Specimens of neoplasms from previous surgery will be used to study specific oncogenes as markers of and as participants in radiation-induced neoplastic transformation. These studies will focus on rearrangements of the ret protooncogene in thyroid neoplasms and the NF2 tumor suppressor gene in neural tumors.

Website: http://commons.cit.nih.gov/crisp3/CRISP.Generate_Ticket

- **Project Title: Tumor Suppressors and Differentiated Thyroid Cancer**

    Principal Investigator & Institution: Eberhardt, Norman L.; Professor; Mayo Clinic Rochester 200 1St St Sw Rochester, Mn 55905

    Timing: Fiscal Year 2000; Project Start 5-JAN-1999; Project End 1-DEC-2001

    Summary: Thyroid malignancies, the most common endocrine cancer, account for >17,000 new cases and 1,200 cancer deaths per year in the U.S. The bulk (70-95%) of these neoplasms are primary thyroid carcinomas of follicular cell origin, including differentiated papillary (PTC) and follicular (FTC), and undifferentiated anaplastic thyroid cancers. In the U.S. incidence rates are PTC > FTC >> anaplastic carcinomas, while morbidity/mortality rates associated with these cancers are anaplastic carcinomas >> FTC >PTC. Evidence for progression from benign follicular adenoma (Fa) > FTC has been observed, while PTC appears to arise de novo. While numerous studies have attempted to define the molecular genetics of differentiated thyroid cancer, virtually all of these studies have suffered from lack of significant specimen numbers, insufficient pathological criteria, or both. We have shown extensive evidence for frequent loss of heterozygosity (LOH) on chromosomes 3p, 10q, 13q and 17p in FTC, but not FA or PTC, suggesting that tumor suppressor genes (TSGs) may be involved in the genesis of FTC. Known TSGs mapping near regions of LOH on chromosomes 3p (VHL and FHIT) and 17p (p53) do not appear to be involved, since mutations of these sequences are rare in FTC. Thus as yet undefined TSGs appears to be involved in the genesis of FTC. In the current studies we will perform a detail molecular genetic study of at least 30 specimen/tumor type of a well defined and stratified population of thyroid cancers, in which extensive clinical records are available. Tumor types will include PTC (grades 1,2 and 3), FTC (minimally and widely invasive, oxyphilic and non-oxyphilic carcinomas) and FA. With this population of tumors we will: (i) perform a comprehensive LOH analysis of all chromosomes arms at a resolution of approximately 10 cM, (ii) refine mapping of regions of significant LOH at a resolution of less than or qual to 2 cM, (iii) analyze candidate TSGs that resides within the refine map locations and (iv) clone potential tumor suppressor genes that reside in locations for which no known TSG candidates have been identified. The molecular genetic profiles will be correlated with the clinical records to assess the significance of the genetic changes on morbidity and mortality. These studies will offer one of the first comprehensive analyses of LOH in any well defined tumor population that can be reconciled with the clinical record and will provide detailed insight into the pathogenesis of thyroid cancer.

Website: http://commons.cit.nih.gov/crisp3/CRISP.Generate_Ticket

- **Project Title: Use of Recombinant Human Thyroid Stimulating Hormone in a Thyroid Cancer Pt**

  Principal Investigator & Institution: Burge, Mark R.; University of New Mexico Albuquerque Albuquerque, Nm 87131

  Timing: Fiscal Year 2000

  Summary: The objective of this study is to use human recombinant human thyroid stimulating hormone, Thyrogen (Genzyme Corporation), an investigational drug, as a compassionate use therapy in a patient with metastatic papillary cancer of the thyroid.

Website: http://commons.cit.nih.gov/crisp3/CRISP.Generate_Ticket

- **Project Title: Demethylation Therapy of Thyroid Carcinoma**

    Principal Investigator & Institution: Ain, Kenneth B.; Internal Medicine; University of Kentucky University Sta Lexington, Ky 40506

    Timing: Fiscal Year 2000; Project Start 4-MAY-2000; Project End 1-MAR-2005

    Summary: (Applicant's Description) Disseminated dedifferentiated thyroid epithelial carcinoma is a terminal disease with no effective systemic treatment or chemotherapy, as a consequence of the loss of the ability to concentrate iodide, rendering it unable to be treated with radioactive iodide. Our translational research efforts aim to restore the therapeutic effectiveness of radioiodine for systemic therapy. Iodide uptake depends upon expression of the human sodium-iodide membrane symporter (hNIS). Chemical agents, differentiation inducers and demethylation agents, have been able to restore lost differentiated functions in a wide variety of other tumor types. Our data show that demethylation agents can restore expression of hNIS mRNA in dedifferentiated human thyroid cancer cell lines and restore iodide uptake. We have shown that this is likely consequent to demethylation of CpG islands of the hNIS gene promoter (or the promoters of thyroid-specific transcription factors) in tumor samples. For this reason, we hypothesize that methylation-induced loss of hNIS gene transcription is reversible by chemical therapy with demethylating agents or differentiation inducers. Such therapy should enable radioiodide treatment of dedifferentiated thyroid cancers. In addition, we have demonstrated that the same mechanism of gene methylation is responsible for loss of expression of E-cadherin, a protein contributing to cell:cell adhesion in human thyroid cancer cells. Restoration of E-cadherin expression may suppress tumor invasion and metastasis, improving the clinical course of thyroid cancer patients. In this way, clinical use of demethylation agents may enhance the effectiveness of therapeutic radioiodine and simultaneously diminish the progression and spread of disease. This proposed patient-oriented research will utilize demethylation agents to restore or enhance radioiodine uptake in thyroid carcinoma metastases of patients previously unresponsive to radioiodine treatment. Pilot trials using known active agents, such as 5-azacytidine, will be supplemented with trials of additional agents defined by cell culture and xenograft studies. Patients with therapeutically-unresponsive dedifferentiated thyroid cancer metastases are often treated with palliative surgical resection of gross tumor. In such patients, fresh tumor samples will be analyzed for hNIS gene methylation and E-cadherin expression and cultured for cell lines. These analyses and in vitro studies will permit targeting of specific agents to individual patients for the purposes of both radioiodine therapy and modulation of tumor progression. Such patient-oriented research will proceed in the context of active mentorship in thyroid oncology and translational research centered on Oncology fellows.

Website: http://commons.cit.nih.gov/crisp3/CRISP.Generate_Ticket

- **Project Title: Establish of Post Chernobyl NIS Thyroid Banks**

  Principal Investigator & Institution: Thomas, Geraldine A.; University of Cambridge Cambridge, England Cambridge,

  Timing: Fiscal Year 2000; Project Start 7-JUL-2000; Project End 0-JUN-2003

  Summary: (Applicant's Description) This project will form an internationally supported collaborative research resource for many groups working on the problems of thyroid cancer which has followed the Chernobyl accident. It is designed to promote collaboration and avoid competition in the use of limited and very valued resources. The four funding organizations involved in the project are the National Institute of Health of the USA, the European Commission, the World Health Organization and the Sasakawa Memorial Health Foundation of Japan. The basis of the project is a collaborative approach to the collection of the tissue from cases of thyroid cancer in the areas around Chernobyl with simultaneous collection of blood samples and basic clinical information. The project has several aims (a) to ensure that the best possible diagnostic service is given to patients, (b) to provide a diagnosis agreed by internationally recognized pathologists. This diagnosis will be made available to research groups from those countries carrying out molecular biological, therapeutic, epidemiological and other studies. (c) to ensure that specimens of thyroid cancer are properly described and sampled, and that materials are available for appropriate research studies (frozen tissue, fixed tissue sections, extracted DNA/RNA and blood samples, together with relevant information), through a protocol agreed by the research organizations involved. The project will provide a valuable research tool for future researchers interested in the mechanism of radiation tumourigenesis of the thyroid following irradiation.

  Website: http://commons.cit.nih.gov/crisp3/CRISP.Generate_Ticket

- **Project Title: General Clinical Research Center**

    Principal Investigator & Institution: Boat, Thomas F.; Director; Children's Hospital Med Ctr (Cincinnati) 3333 Burnet Ave Cincinnati, Oh 45229

    Timing: Fiscal Year 2000; Project Start 0-DEC-1993; Project End 0-NOV-2001

    Summary: This is a proposal for the renewal of a multi-categorical General Clinical Research Center at the Children's and University Hospitals. Major areas of research include: 1. Pediatric Liver Disease. Studies are defining the pathophysiology and treatment of new inborn errors of bile acid metabolism and peroxisomal disorders and the pathogenesis of bone disease and growth failure in cholestatic liver disease. 2. Bone Health. Studies will examine the effect of maternal age during lactation on bone demineralization and the value of progestins in ameliorating the loss. Studies will evaluate the role of calcium supplementation on bone accretion in prepubertal children, the role of exercise in bone accretion in preschoolers and the pathogenesis and management of bone disease in juvenile rheumatoid arthritis. 3. Cancer. Using resources available through a proposed Tissue Procurement Facility supported by the GCRC, basic science and clinical investigators will obtain tumors for investigations of the cell biology and molecular mechanisms of malignancies. Studies will investigate thyroid cancer, neural tumors, breast cancer, and the APC and Bloom's Syndrome genes. 4. Gaucher Disease. Despite the availability of enzyme research for Gaucher Disease, disability from bone disease persists. Studies will evaluate the potential value of bisphosphonates as an adjunct to enzyme replacement for the treatment of bone disease in Gaucher Disease. 5. Cystic Fibrosis. Studies are defining the safety of a replication-deficient recombinant adenovirus construct to deliver the CF transmembrane conductance gene to the nasal epithelium. 6. Cholesterol Synthesis. Studies are evaluating the potential effect of the cholesterol content in breast milk or infant formulae and cholesterol synthesis rates to determine if early exposure to cholesterol in the human infant may have an "imprinting" effect on cholesterol synthesis.

    Website: http://commons.cit.nih.gov/crisp3/CRISP.Generate_Ticket

- **Project Title: Glucose Homeostasis in Aging**

    Principal Investigator & Institution: Convit, Antonio; New York University School of Medicine 550 1St Ave New York, Ny 10016

    Timing: Fiscal Year 2000

    Summary: This Phase I clinical trial attempts to determine the qualitative and quantitative toxicities of topotecan when given by prolonged infusion in combination with radiation therapy and their maximally tolerated dose in combination. It also attempts to document the degree of antitumor activity observed. Eligible tumor types, include but are not limited to, nonsmall cell lung, esophageal cancer, melanoma, mesothelioma, and thyroid cancer. The patients must be eligible for chest radiation.

Website: http://commons.cit.nih.gov/crisp3/CRISP.Generate_Ticket

- **Project Title: Molecular-Genetic Analysis of 3p14 Genomic Stability**

Principal Investigator & Institution: Drabkin, Harry A.; Professor; Medicine; University of Colorado Hlth Sciences Ctr 4200 E 9Th Ave Denver, Co 80262

Timing: Fiscal Year 2000; Project Start 4-AUG-1998; Project End 0-APR-2002

Summary: (Adapted from the Investigator's Abstract): The hereditary renal carcinoma 3;8 translocation has been the source of considerable interest among cancer geneticists and a long-term goal of this laboratory. The pattern of disease is one of classic hereditary cancer with autosomal dominant inheritance, multifocal early onset renal cancer and less frequently, thyroid cancer. The investigators were the first to clone the 3p14 translocation breakpoint. Their subsequent investigations identified homozygous deletions in various carcinoma cell lines involving a region approximately 150 kb telomeric to the t(3;8) breakpoint. This region coincides with FRA3B, the most inducible fragile site in the genome. Whether or not the deletions involving FRA3B result solely from genomic instability, or are biologically selected, is an important question, given the high frequency of 3p loss in a variety of malignant diseases. While Ohta et al. identified a 3p14 gene, FHIT, spanning the 3;8 breakpoint, its role as a tumor suppressor has been seriously questioned. The investigators have discovered that the 3;8 translocation results in a fusion transcript between a novel gene, TRC8, and FHIT. The TRC8 gene is suggested to be a membrane receptor with partial similarity to Drosophila patched, the human homologue of which is responsible for the hereditary basal cell carcinoma syndrome. With regard to the distinct 3p14 deletion region, the investigators have obtained evidence for additional non-FHIT transcripts and have identified a cell line, CC19, with ongoing spontaneous deletions in FRA3B which exhibit tumorigenic differences. This system provides an ideal model to investigate the tumorigenic role of FHIT and other putative genes. The investigators propose, therefore, two main areas of investigation: 1) The further characterization of TRC8 including a mutational analysis of renal and thyroid carcinomas; development of antibodies for the subcellular localization of normal and rearranged products; transfection experiments to functionally characterize the TRC8, TRC8-FHIT and FHIT-TRC8 products. 2) To clarify the role of 3p14 deletions in cancer, they will examine the tumorigenesis of CC19 subclones with and without deletions affecting FHIT exons. If consistent correlations between deletions and tumorigenic variation can be obtained, they will perform transfection experiments with FHIT to confirm this activity. If non-FHIT coding regions are suggested to have tumor suppressor activity they will be further characterized.

Website: http://commons.cit.nih.gov/crisp3/CRISP.Generate_Ticket

- **Project Title: Protein Kinase C And Thyroid Cell Apoptosis**

  Principal Investigator & Institution: Knauf, Jeffrey A.; Internal Medicine; University of Cincinnati 2624 Clifton Ave Cincinnati, Oh 45221

  Timing: Fiscal Year 2000; Project Start 1-APR-2000; Project End 0-NOV-2002

  Summary: (taken from the application) In 1997, there were an estimated 16,100 new cases of thyroid cancer in the United States. Cancer is not simply a proliferation process, but the manifestation of an imbalance between cell growth and cell death. It is likely that for a tumor clone to progress the apoptotic program must be successfully disabled. In support of this paradigm, we have isolated a chimeric and truncated mutant of PKC-epsilon (Tr-PKC-epsilon), the gene for which was amplified and rearranged in a thyroid cancer cell line. When transfected into PCCL3 cells (a well-differentiated rat thyroid cell line) Tr-PKC-epsilon inhibits activation-induced translocation of the wild-type isozyme, resulting in protection of cells from apoptosis. This is accompanied by a marked impairment in p53 stabilization, which may be in part due to elevated levels of MDM2. These findings point to a role for PKC-epsilon in apoptosis signaling pathways in thyroid cells, and suggest that disruptions in PKC-epsilon function may be involved in thyroid tumorigenesis, possibly by altering the cellular response to DNA damage. In support of this we have found that in 75-85% of thyroid carcinomas there were dramatic changes in the level and/or subcellular distribution of PKC-epsilon compared to corresponding normal thyroid tissue. The following Specific Aims are proposed: (1) We will use an inducible expression system to achieve selective activation of either PKC-epsilon or the constitutively activated mutant PKC-epsilon-A159F and to determine whether this alone can initiate an apoptotic program, that can be blocked by Tr-PKC-epsilon. (2) We will explore whether PKC-epsilon activation interferes with phosphorylation, stabilization, and other post-translational modifications of p53 and MDM-2. (3) We will manipulate the function of the isozyme in thyroid follicular cells of transgenic mice, by targeting expression of either PKC-epsilon, PDK-epsilon-A159F, or the dominant negative inhibitor Tr-PKC-epsilon. Effects on thyroid cell apoptosis in vivo will then be studied in mice exposed to external radiation to the thyroid bed. (4) We will determine if the observed changes in expression and distribution of PKC-epsilon in thyroid cancers are due to somatically-acquired structural defects in the PKC-epsilon gene, or to epigenetic events. For tumor clones to expand, they must not only exhibit unrestrained stimulation to proliferate, but must also disable essential protection circuits that trigger apoptosis. We propose that PKC-epsilon is part of this defensive strategy, and that this can be subverted during tumorigenesis, or perhaps modulated during adaptive responses such as goiter involution, or thyroid remodeling.

Website: http://commons.cit.nih.gov/crisp3/CRISP.Generate_Ticket

- **Project Title: Regulation of the Sodium/Iodide Symporter in Breast**

    Principal Investigator & Institution: Brent, Gregory A.; Professor; Medicine; University of California Los Angeles 10920 Wilshire Blvd., Suite 1200 Los Angeles, Ca 90024

    Timing: Fiscal Year 2001; Project Start 2-JAN-2001; Project End 1-DEC-2004

    Summary: (Adapted from the applicant's abstract) In the lactating mammary gland, iodide is concentrated up to 36-fold in milk compared with the plasma iodide concentration, due to stimulation of the sodium/iodide symporter (NIS). Some hormone-dependent breast cancers also concentrate iodide, up to 7-fold, but iodide uptake in breast cancer must be enhanced to make radioiodine treatment possible, analogous to the TSH stimulation required for uptake of radioiodine into thyroid cancer. All-trans retinoic acid (RA) treatment stimulates iodide uptake, MS mRNA, and MS protein in MCF-7 cells, an estrogen receptor (ER) positive human breast cancer cell line, in a time and dose dependent fashion. No RA-induction of iodide uptake is seen in an ER-negative breast cancer cell line, MDA-MB 231, or a normal breast-derived cell line, MCF-12A. An in vitro clonogenic assay demonstrated selective toxicity of radioiodine following RA stimulation of MCF-7 cells. MCF-12A cells have abundant MS protein, but no functional iodide uptake. MS regulation differs significantly in the breast compared to the thyroid, and differs in normal breast and breast cancer cell lines. We propose to study the regulation of iodide transport in breast cancer cell lines compared to normal breast and thyroid cell lines, with the goals of optimzing iodide uptake and selectively targeting breast cancer cells. Specific aims include: 1. Determine the mechanism of RA-mediated transcriptional regulation of the NIS gene in breast-derived cells utilizing selective retinoid agonists and cell lines with a range of endogenous RAR and RXR expression. 2. To determine the characteristics of NIS protein expression, subcellular localization, and kinetics that are associated with maximal function of NIS in breast-derived cell lines and those features that distinguish functional iodide uptake among cell lines that express NIS protein. 3. Utilize an in vitro model to optimize RA-stimulated radiation-mediated cell killing in breast cancer cells. 4. Develop in vivo models to determine the efficacy and specificity of RA-stimulated iodide uptake into breast cancer and determine the influence of enhancers and radiation sensitizers. RA raioiodide uptake may be useful for diagnosis and treatment of some differentiated breast cancer.

Website: http://commons.cit.nih.gov/crisp3/CRISP.Generate_Ticket

- **Project Title: Simplified Low Iodine Diet for I 131 Radioiodine Diagnostic Imaging**

    Principal Investigator & Institution: Lee, Stephanie; New England Medical Center Hospitals 750 Washington St Boston, Ma 02111

    Timing: Fiscal Year 2000

    Summary: Radioactive iodine is used for the diagnosis of distant and local metastases of thyroid cancer and therapy of thyrotoxicosis and thyroid cancer. Because of the high iodine content of the American diet, the efficacy of radioiodine is diminished unless that patient is placed on a strict low iodine diet. This diet which consists of freshly prepared meals and homemade breads and pastas is nearly impossible to follow with the American dietary habits of eating in restaurants and using convenience foods. After review of the iodine content of currently available foods, the objective of this study is to develop and test a convenient and palatable out-patient diet to decrease iodine intake and excretion to less than 50mcg/24hrs in normal volunteers and patients undergoing routine radioactive iodine diagnostic scanning or therapy for thyrotoxicosis and thyroid cancer.

    Website: http://commons.cit.nih.gov/crisp3/CRISP.Generate_Ticket

- **Project Title: Structure/Function Relationships of Human Thyrotropin**

    Principal Investigator & Institution: Weintraub, Bruce D.; Chief Scientific Officer; Medicine; University of Maryland Balt Prof School Professional Schools Baltimore, Md 21201

    Timing: Fiscal Year 2000; Project Start 1-SEP-1998; Project End 1-AUG-2001

Summary: The objective of this proposal is the elucidation of the structure- function relationships of human thyrotropin (hTSH) and its receptor by developing and characterizing the action of novel analogs with enhanced binding affinity, in vitro and in vivo biological activity (superactive analogs). There are extensive studies of functional domains of gonadotropins but only limited studies of those in TSH, primarily from our laboratory, which show significant differences in structure-function relationships. Moreover, until our recent observations, there had not been reports for any glycoprotein hormone or any member of the cystine knot growth factor superfamily of such analogs with major increases in receptor binding affinity or in vitro bioactivity. We have initiated the design of superactive analogs based on evolutionary considerations, homology comparison of sequences from various species, and homology modeling of hTSH. The first generation of superactive hTSH analogs displayed up to 1,000-fold increase in potency and 2-fold increased maximal response. To design a second generation of even more potent analogs we will selectively introduce clusters of charged residues, present in homologous hormones, within the peripheral loops of hTSH, separately and in various combinations. In the current proposal we will: 1) perform systematic multidomain mutagenesis in the peripheral hairpin loops of both hTSH subunits to optimize the potency and efficacy of the analogs; 2) express and purify large amounts of the most active analogs and characterize their biochemical and biological properties; 3) attempt to determine the areas of the hTSH receptor that interact with the positively charged residues within the loops of hTSH superactive analogs; 4) test whether site-specific removal of sialic acid will increase the receptor binding and in vitro activity of selected hTSH analogs. These studies should provide novel insights into structure-function relationships of TSH and a novel approach to the study of TSH receptor activation. Highly active recombinant hTSH analogs should be of great value in several in vitro applications related to receptor binding or activation and should have improved therapeutic benefit in stimulating 131I uptake and thyroglobulin secretion in patients with thyroid cancer and nontoxic goiter. High affinity hTSH analogs may also have unique capabilities for novel therapies of thyroid cancer involving targeted delivery of radionuclides, toxins, tumor suppressor genes or the sodium/iodide symporter gene. Moreover, their design provides a rational strategy for the development of similar analogs for other members of the cystine know growth factor superfamily. Finally, the public health importance of this proposal is underscored by the large number of new cases of unusually aggressive childhood thyroid cancer detected in Europe because of the Chernobyl accident and of new adult cases expected in the U.S. because of nuclear testing in Nevada in the 1950's.

Website: http://commons.cit.nih.gov/crisp3/CRISP.Generate_Ticket

E-Journals: PubMed Central[27]

PubMed Central (PMC) is a digital archive of life sciences journal literature developed and managed by the National Center for Biotechnology Information (NCBI) at the U.S. National Library of Medicine (NLM).[28] Access to this growing archive of e-journals is free and unrestricted.[29] To search, go to **http://www.pubmedcentral.nih.gov/index.html#search**, and type "thyroid cancer" (or synonyms) into the search box. This search gives you access to full-text articles. The following is a sample of items found for thyroid cancer in the PubMed Central database:

- **A 1.5-Megabase Yeast Artificial Chromosome Contig from Human Chromosome 10q11.2 Connecting Three Genetic Loci (RET, D10S94, and D10S102) Closely Linked to the MEN2A Locus** by TC Lairmore, S Dou, JR Howe, D Chi, K Carlson, R Veile, SK Mishra, SA Wells, Jr, and H Donis-Keller; 1993 January 15
  http://www.pubmedcentral.nih.gov/articlerender.fcgi?rendertype=abstract&artid=45689

- **A dimeric mutant of human pancreatic ribonuclease with selective cytotoxicity toward malignant cells** by Renata Piccoli, Sonia Di Gaetano, Claudia De Lorenzo, Michela Grauso, Carmen Monaco, Daniela Spalletti-Cernia, Paolo Laccetti, Jaroslav Cinatl, Josef Matousek, and Giuseppe D'Alessio; 1999 July 6
  http://www.pubmedcentral.nih.gov/articlerender.fcgi?artid=22136

- **Adenovirus-mediated suppression of HMGI(Y) protein synthesis as potential therapy of human malignant neoplasias** by Stefania Scala, Giuseppe Portella, Monica Fedele, Gennaro Chiappetta, and Alfredo Fusco; 2000 April 11
  http://www.pubmedcentral.nih.gov/articlerender.fcgi?artid=18219

- **Characterization of an Inversion on the Long Arm of Chromosome 10 Juxtaposing D10S170 and RET and Creating the Oncogenic Sequence**

---

[27] Adapted from the National Library of Medicine: **http://www.pubmedcentral.nih.gov/about/intro.html**.
[28] With PubMed Central, NCBI is taking the lead in preservation and maintenance of open access to electronic literature, just as NLM has done for decades with printed biomedical literature. PubMed Central aims to become a world-class library of the digital age.
[29] The value of PubMed Central, in addition to its role as an archive, lies the availability of data from diverse sources stored in a common format in a single repository. Many journals already have online publishing operations, and there is a growing tendency to publish material online only, to the exclusion of print.

RET/PTC by MA Pierotti, M Santoro, RB Jenkins, G Sozzi, I Bongarzone, M Grieco, N Monzini, M Miozzo, MA Herrmann, A Fusco, ID Hay, GD Porta, and G Vecchio; 1992 March 1
http://www.pubmedcentral.nih.gov/articlerender.fcgi?rendertype=abstract&artid=48503

- **Development of medullary thyroid carcinoma in transgenic mice expressing the RET protooncogene altered by a multiple endocrine neoplasia type 2A mutation** by Francine-Marie Michiels, Sophie Chappuis, Bernard Caillou, Andrea Pasini, Monique Talbot, Roger Monier, Gilbert M. Lenoir, Jean Feunteun, and Marc Billaud; 1997 April 1
http://www.pubmedcentral.nih.gov/articlerender.fcgi?artid=20369

- **Fine-needle aspiration biopsy of the thyroid** by Kenneth C. Suen; 2002 September 3
http://www.pubmedcentral.nih.gov/articlerender.fcgi?artid=121968

- **Gene expression in papillary thyroid carcinoma reveals highly consistent profiles** by Ying Huang, Manju Prasad, William J. Lemon, Heather Hampel, Fred A. Wright, Karl Kornacker, Virginia LiVolsi, Wendy Frankel, Richard T. Kloos, Charis Eng, Natalia S. Pellegata, and Albert de la Chapelle; 2001 December 18
http://www.pubmedcentral.nih.gov/articlerender.fcgi?artid=64980

The National Library of Medicine: PubMed

One of the quickest and most comprehensive ways to find academic studies in both English and other languages is to use PubMed, maintained by the National Library of Medicine. The advantage of PubMed over previously mentioned sources is that it covers a greater number of domestic and foreign references. It is also free to the public.[30] If the publisher has a Web site that offers full text of its journals, PubMed will provide links to that site, as well as to sites offering other related data. User registration, a subscription fee, or some other type of fee may be required to access the full text of articles in some journals.

---

[30] PubMed was developed by the National Center for Biotechnology Information (NCBI) at the National Library of Medicine (NLM) at the National Institutes of Health (NIH). The PubMed database was developed in conjunction with publishers of biomedical literature as a search tool for accessing literature citations and linking to full-text journal articles at Web sites of participating publishers. Publishers that participate in PubMed supply NLM with their citations electronically prior to or at the time of publication.

To generate your own bibliography of studies dealing with thyroid cancer, simply go to the PubMed Web site at **www.ncbi.nlm.nih.gov/pubmed**. Type "thyroid cancer" (or synonyms) into the search box, and click "Go." The following is the type of output you can expect from PubMed for "thyroid cancer" (hyperlinks lead to article summaries):

- **123 I as a diagnostic tracer in the management of thyroid cancer.**
  Author(s): Kalinyak JE.
  Source: Nuclear Medicine Communications. 2002 June; 23(6): 509-11. No Abstract Available.
  http://www.ncbi.nlm.nih.gov:80/entrez/query.fcgi?cmd=Retrieve&db=PubMed&list_uids=12029204&dopt=Abstract

- **A thyroid-specific far-upstream enhancer in the human sodium/iodide symporter gene requires pax-8 binding and cyclic adenosine 3',5'-monophosphate response element-like sequence binding proteins for full activity and is differentially regulated in normal and thyroid cancer cells.**
  Author(s): Taki K, Kogai T, Kanamoto Y, Hershman JM, Brent GA.
  Source: Molecular Endocrinology (Baltimore, Md.). 2002 October; 16(10): 2266-82.
  http://www.ncbi.nlm.nih.gov:80/entrez/query.fcgi?cmd=Retrieve&db=PubMed&list_uids=12351692&dopt=Abstract

- **Aberrant localization of beta-catenin correlates with overexpression of its target gene in human papillary thyroid cancer.**
  Author(s): Ishigaki K, Namba H, Nakashima M, Nakayama T, Mitsutake N, Hayashi T, Maeda S, Ichinose M, Kanematsu T, Yamashita S.
  Source: The Journal of Clinical Endocrinology and Metabolism. 2002 July; 87(7): 3433-40.
  http://www.ncbi.nlm.nih.gov:80/entrez/query.fcgi?cmd=Retrieve&db=PubMed&list_uids=12107263&dopt=Abstract

- **Ablation of thyroid residues with 30 mCi (131)I: a comparison in thyroid cancer patients prepared with recombinant human TSH or thyroid hormone withdrawal.**
  Author(s): Pacini F, Molinaro E, Castagna MG, Lippi F, Ceccarelli C, Agate L, Elisei R, Pinchera A.
  Source: The Journal of Clinical Endocrinology and Metabolism. 2002 September; 87(9): 4063-8.
  http://www.ncbi.nlm.nih.gov:80/entrez/query.fcgi?cmd=Retrieve&db=PubMed&list_uids=12213846&dopt=Abstract

- **Benign thyroid disease and dietary factors in thyroid cancer: a case-control study in Kuwait.**
  Author(s): Memon A, Varghese A, Suresh A.
  Source: British Journal of Cancer. 2002 June 5; 86(11): 1745-50.
  http://www.ncbi.nlm.nih.gov:80/entrez/query.fcgi?cmd=Retrieve&db=PubMed&list_uids=12087461&dopt=Abstract

- **Chemo-radionuclide therapy for thyroid cancer: initial experimental study with cultured cells.**
  Author(s): Misaki T, Iwata M, Iida Y, Kasagi K, Konishi J.
  Source: Ann Nucl Med. 2002 September; 16(6): 403-8.
  http://www.ncbi.nlm.nih.gov:80/entrez/query.fcgi?cmd=Retrieve&db=PubMed&list_uids=12416579&dopt=Abstract

- **Cholecystokinin-B/Gastrin receptor-targeting peptides for staging and therapy of medullary thyroid cancer and other cholecystokinin-B receptor-expressing malignancies.**
  Author(s): Behr TM, Behe MP.
  Source: Semin Nucl Med. 2002 April; 32(2): 97-109. Review.
  http://www.ncbi.nlm.nih.gov:80/entrez/query.fcgi?cmd=Retrieve&db=PubMed&list_uids=11965605&dopt=Abstract

- **Clinical impact of retinoids in redifferentiation therapy of advanced thyroid cancer: final results of a pilot study.**
  Author(s): Simon D, Korber C, Krausch M, Segering J, Groth P, Gorges R, Grunwald F, Muller-Gartner HW, Schmutzler C, Kohrle J, Roher HD, Reiners C.
  Source: European Journal of Nuclear Medicine and Molecular Imaging. 2002 June; 29(6): 775-82.
  http://www.ncbi.nlm.nih.gov:80/entrez/query.fcgi?cmd=Retrieve&db=PubMed&list_uids=12029551&dopt=Abstract

- **Clinical significance of elevated level of serum antithyroglobulin antibody in patients with differentiated thyroid cancer after thyroid ablation.**
  Author(s): Chung JK, Park YJ, Kim TY, So Y, Kim SK, Park DJ, Lee DS, Lee MC, Cho BY.
  Source: Clinical Endocrinology. 2002 August; 57(2): 215-21.
  http://www.ncbi.nlm.nih.gov:80/entrez/query.fcgi?cmd=Retrieve&db=PubMed&list_uids=12153600&dopt=Abstract

- **Comparison of (123)I and (131)I for whole-body imaging in thyroid cancer.**
  Author(s): Sarkar SD, Kalapparambath TP, Palestro CJ.
  Source: Journal of Nuclear Medicine : Official Publication, Society of Nuclear Medicine. 2002 May; 43(5): 632-4.
  http://www.ncbi.nlm.nih.gov:80/entrez/query.fcgi?cmd=Retrieve&db=PubMed&list_uids=11994526&dopt=Abstract

- **Complementary role of 18F-fluorodeoxyglucose positron emission tomography and 131I scan in the follow-up of post-therapy differentiated thyroid cancer.**
  Author(s): Hsu CH, Liu RS, Wu CH, Chen SM, Shih LS.
  Source: J Formos Med Assoc. 2002 July; 101(7): 459-67.
  http://www.ncbi.nlm.nih.gov:80/entrez/query.fcgi?cmd=Retrieve&db=PubMed&list_uids=12353337&dopt=Abstract

- **Complications of neck dissection for thyroid cancer.**
  Author(s): Cheah WK, Arici C, Ituarte PH, Siperstein AE, Duh QY, Clark OH.
  Source: World Journal of Surgery. 2002 August; 26(8): 1013-6.
  http://www.ncbi.nlm.nih.gov:80/entrez/query.fcgi?cmd=Retrieve&db=PubMed&list_uids=12045861&dopt=Abstract

- **Contralateral papillary thyroid cancer-high incidence in therapeutic completion thyroidectomy.**
  Author(s): Gemsenjager E, Heitz PU.
  Source: Thyroid : Official Journal of the American Thyroid Association. 2002 April; 12(4): 345-6. No Abstract Available.
  http://www.ncbi.nlm.nih.gov:80/entrez/query.fcgi?cmd=Retrieve&db=PubMed&list_uids=12034063&dopt=Abstract

- **Contribution of an Anti-CEA Fab' scan in the detection of medullary thyroid cancer.**
  Author(s): Malamitsi J, Kosmidis PA, Papadopoulos S, Petounis A, Linos DA.
  Source: Clinical Nuclear Medicine. 2002 June; 27(6): 447-8. No Abstract Available.
  http://www.ncbi.nlm.nih.gov:80/entrez/query.fcgi?cmd=Retrieve&db=PubMed&list_uids=12045444&dopt=Abstract

- **Current controversies in the mnnagement of pediatric patients with well-differentiated nonmedullary thyroid cancer: a review.**
  Author(s): Hung W, Sarlis NJ.
  Source: Thyroid : Official Journal of the American Thyroid Association. 2002 August; 12(8): 683-702.
  http://www.ncbi.nlm.nih.gov:80/entrez/query.fcgi?cmd=Retrieve&db=PubMed&list_uids=12225637&dopt=Abstract

- **Current national health insurance policies for thyroid cancer prophylactic surgery in the United States.**
  Author(s): Dackiw AP, Kuerer HM, Clark OH.
  Source: World Journal of Surgery. 2002 August; 26(8): 903-6.
  http://www.ncbi.nlm.nih.gov:80/entrez/query.fcgi?cmd=Retrieve&db=PubMed&list_uids=12045864&dopt=Abstract

- **Cytotoxic effects of carboplatinum and epirubicin in the setting of an elevated serum thyrotropin for advanced poorly differentiated thyroid cancer.**
  Author(s): Santini F, Bottici V, Elisei R, Montanelli L, Mazzeo S, Basolo F, Pinchera A, Pacini F.
  Source: The Journal of Clinical Endocrinology and Metabolism. 2002 September; 87(9): 4160-5.
  http://www.ncbi.nlm.nih.gov:80/entrez/query.fcgi?cmd=Retrieve&db=PubMed&list_uids=12213865&dopt=Abstract

- **Determination of galectin-3 messenger ribonucleic Acid overexpression in papillary thyroid cancer by quantitative reverse transcription-polymerase chain reaction.**
  Author(s): Bernet VJ, Anderson J, Vaishnav Y, Solomon B, Adair CF, Saji M, Burman KD, Burch HB, Ringel MD.
  Source: The Journal of Clinical Endocrinology and Metabolism. 2002 October; 87(10): 4792-6.
  http://www.ncbi.nlm.nih.gov:80/entrez/query.fcgi?cmd=Retrieve&db=PubMed&list_uids=12364475&dopt=Abstract

- **Diabetes and infarcted papillary thyroid cancer.**
  Author(s): Haddad FH, Malkawi OM, Omari AA, Izzat AS, Khassrof HM, Faiad LM, Okla AL, Jamil AN.
  Source: Saudi Med J. 2002 April; 23(4): 467-70.
  http://www.ncbi.nlm.nih.gov:80/entrez/query.fcgi?cmd=Retrieve&db=PubMed&list_uids=11953778&dopt=Abstract

- **Differentiated thyroid cancer presenting as distant metastases.**
  Author(s): Mishra A, Mishra SK, Das BK, Pradhan PK.
  Source: The European Journal of Surgery = Acta Chirurgica. 2002; 168(5): 305-9. No Abstract Available.
  http://www.ncbi.nlm.nih.gov:80/entrez/query.fcgi?cmd=Retrieve&db=PubMed&list_uids=12375614&dopt=Abstract

- **Endoscopic ultrasonography in patients with thyroid cancer: its usefulness and limitations for evaluating esophagopharyngeal invasion.**
  Author(s): Koike E, Yamashita H, Noguchi S, Ohshima A, Yamashita H, Watanabe S, Uchino S, Arita T, Kuroki S, Tanaka M.
  Source: Endoscopy. 2002 June; 34(6): 457-60.
  http://www.ncbi.nlm.nih.gov:80/entrez/query.fcgi?cmd=Retrieve&db=PubMed&list_uids=12048627&dopt=Abstract

- **Establishment and characterization of OCUT-1, an undifferentiated thyroid cancer cell line expressing high level of telomerase.**
  Author(s): Ogisawa K, Onoda N, Ishikawa T, Takenaka C, Inaba M, Ogawa Y, Chung KH.
  Source: Journal of Surgical Oncology. 2002 August; 80(4): 197-203.
  http://www.ncbi.nlm.nih.gov:80/entrez/query.fcgi?cmd=Retrieve&db=PubMed&list_uids=12210034&dopt=Abstract

- **Expansion of Microsatellite in the Thyroid Hormone Receptor-alpha1 Gene Linked to Increased Receptor Expression and Less Aggressive Thyroid Cancer.**
  Author(s): Onda M, Li D, Suzuki S, Nakamura I, Takenoshita S, Brogren CH, Stampanoni S, Rampino N.
  Source: Clinical Cancer Research : an Official Journal of the American Association for Cancer Research. 2002 September; 8(9): 2870-4.
  http://www.ncbi.nlm.nih.gov:80/entrez/query.fcgi?cmd=Retrieve&db=PubMed&list_uids=12231529&dopt=Abstract

- **Familial nonmedullary thyroid cancer.**
  Author(s): Alsanea O.
  Source: Curr Treat Options Oncol. 2000 October; 1(4): 345-51. Review.
  http://www.ncbi.nlm.nih.gov:80/entrez/query.fcgi?cmd=Retrieve&db=PubMed&list_uids=12061376&dopt=Abstract

- **Follow-up of differentiated thyroid cancer.**
  Author(s): Pacini F.

Source: European Journal of Nuclear Medicine and Molecular Imaging. 2002 August; 29(Supplement 2): S492-6.
http://www.ncbi.nlm.nih.gov:80/entrez/query.fcgi?cmd=Retrieve&db=PubMed&list_uids=12192551&dopt=Abstract

- **Genetic Changes in Chromosomes 1p and 17p in Thyroid Cancer Progression.**
  Author(s): Kleer CG, Bryant BR, Giordano TJ, Sobel M, Merino MJ.
  Source: Endocr Pathol. 2000 Summer; 11(2): 137-143.
  http://www.ncbi.nlm.nih.gov:80/entrez/query.fcgi?cmd=Retrieve&db=PubMed&list_uids=12114819&dopt=Abstract

- **Genetic disregulation of gene coding tumor necrosis factor alpha receptors (TNF alpha Rs) in follicular thyroid cancer--preliminary report.**
  Author(s): Zubelewicz B, Muc-Wierzgon M, Wierzgon J, Romanowski W, Mazurek U, Wilczok T, Podwinska E.
  Source: J Biol Regul Homeost Agents. 2002 April-June; 16(2): 98-104.
  http://www.ncbi.nlm.nih.gov:80/entrez/query.fcgi?cmd=Retrieve&db=PubMed&list_uids=12144133&dopt=Abstract

- **Genetic events in the evolution of thyroid cancer.**
  Author(s): Freeman J, Carroll C, Asa S, Ezzat S.
  Source: The Journal of Otolaryngology. 2002 August; 31(4): 202-6.
  http://www.ncbi.nlm.nih.gov:80/entrez/query.fcgi?cmd=Retrieve&db=PubMed&list_uids=12240753&dopt=Abstract

- **Genome-Wide Appraisal of Thyroid Cancer Progression.**
  Author(s): Wreesmann VB, Ghossein RA, Patel SG, Harris CP, Schnaser EA, Shaha AR, Tuttle RM, Shah JP, Rao PH, Singh B.
  Source: American Journal of Pathology. 2002 November; 161(5): 1549-1556.
  http://www.ncbi.nlm.nih.gov:80/entrez/query.fcgi?cmd=Retrieve&db=PubMed&list_uids=12414503&dopt=Abstract

- **Gonadal damage from 131I therapy for thyroid cancer.**
  Author(s): Mazzaferri EL.
  Source: Clinical Endocrinology. 2002 September; 57(3): 313-4. No Abstract Available.
  http://www.ncbi.nlm.nih.gov:80/entrez/query.fcgi?cmd=Retrieve&db=PubMed&list_uids=12201822&dopt=Abstract

- **High resolution loss of heterozygosity mapping of 17p13 in thyroid cancer: Hurthle cell carcinomas exhibit a small 411-kilobase common region of allelic imbalance, probably containing a novel tumor suppressor gene.**
  Author(s): Farrand K, Delahunt B, Wang XL, McIver B, Hay ID, Goellner JR, Eberhardt NL, Grebe SK.
  Source: The Journal of Clinical Endocrinology and Metabolism. 2002 October; 87(10): 4715-21.
  http://www.ncbi.nlm.nih.gov:80/entrez/query.fcgi?cmd=Retrieve&db=PubMed&list_uids=12364463&dopt=Abstract

- **Highly sensitive serum thyroglobulin and circulating thyroglobulin mRNA evaluations in the management of patients with differentiated thyroid cancer in apparent remission.**
  Author(s): Fugazzola L, Mihalich A, Persani L, Cerutti N, Reina M, Bonomi M, Ponti E, Mannavola D, Giammona E, Vannucchi G, di Blasio AM, Beck-Peccoz P.
  Source: The Journal of Clinical Endocrinology and Metabolism. 2002 July; 87(7): 3201-8.
  http://www.ncbi.nlm.nih.gov:80/entrez/query.fcgi?cmd=Retrieve&db=PubMed&list_uids=12107225&dopt=Abstract

- **High-sensitive 2(nd) generation thyroglobulin immunoradiometric assay. Clinical application in differentiated thyroid cancer management.**
  Author(s): Giovanella L, Ceriani L, Garancini S.
  Source: Q J Nucl Med. 2002 December; 46(4): 319-322.
  http://www.ncbi.nlm.nih.gov:80/entrez/query.fcgi?cmd=Retrieve&db=PubMed&list_uids=12411872&dopt=Abstract

- **High-sensitivity human thyroglobulin (hTG) immunoradiometric assay in the follow-up of patients with differentiated thyroid cancer.**
  Author(s): Giovanella L, Ceriani L.
  Source: Clinical Chemistry and Laboratory Medicine : Cclm / Fescc. 2002 May; 40(5): 480-4.
  http://www.ncbi.nlm.nih.gov:80/entrez/query.fcgi?cmd=Retrieve&db=PubMed&list_uids=12113292&dopt=Abstract

- **Impact of cervical lymph node dissection on serum TG and the course of disease in TG-positive, radioactive iodine whole body scan-negative recurrent/persistent papillary thyroid cancer.**

Author(s): Alzahrani AS, Raef H, Sultan A, Al Sobhi S, Ingemansson S, Ahmed M, Al Mahfouz A.
Source: J Endocrinol Invest. 2002 June; 25(6): 526-31.
http://www.ncbi.nlm.nih.gov:80/entrez/query.fcgi?cmd=Retrieve&db=PubMed&list_uids=12109624&dopt=Abstract

- **Impact of nodal metastases on prognosis in patients with well-differentiated thyroid cancer.**
  Author(s): Beasley NJ, Lee J, Eski S, Walfish P, Witterick I, Freeman JL.
  Source: Archives of Otolaryngology--Head & Neck Surgery. 2002 July; 128(7): 825-8.
  http://www.ncbi.nlm.nih.gov:80/entrez/query.fcgi?cmd=Retrieve&db=PubMed&list_uids=12117344&dopt=Abstract

- **Impact of timing on completion thyroidectomy for thyroid cancer.**
  Author(s): Tan MP, Agarwal G, Reeve TS, Barraclough BH, Delbridge LW.
  Source: The British Journal of Surgery. 2002 June; 89(6): 802-4.
  http://www.ncbi.nlm.nih.gov:80/entrez/query.fcgi?cmd=Retrieve&db=PubMed&list_uids=12027996&dopt=Abstract

- **Importance of lymph node metastases in follicular thyroid cancer.**
  Author(s): Witte J, Goretzki PE, Dieken J, Simon D, Roher HD.
  Source: World Journal of Surgery. 2002 August; 26(8): 1017-22.
  http://www.ncbi.nlm.nih.gov:80/entrez/query.fcgi?cmd=Retrieve&db=PubMed&list_uids=12045860&dopt=Abstract

- **Improved planning of radioiodine therapy for thyroid cancer.**
  Author(s): Medvedec M.
  Source: Journal of Nuclear Medicine : Official Publication, Society of Nuclear Medicine. 2002 May; 43(5): 714; Discussion 714. No Abstract Available.
  http://www.ncbi.nlm.nih.gov:80/entrez/query.fcgi?cmd=Retrieve&db=PubMed&list_uids=11994536&dopt=Abstract

- **Incidence of thyroid cancer in adults recorded by French cancer registries (1978-1997).**
  Author(s): Colonna M, Grosclaude P, Remontet L, Schvartz C, Mace-Lesech J, Velten M, Guizard A, Tretarre B, Buemi A, Arveux P, Esteve J.

Source: European Journal of Cancer (Oxford, England : 1990). 2002 September; 38(13): 1762.
http://www.ncbi.nlm.nih.gov:80/entrez/query.fcgi?cmd=Retrieve&db=PubMed&list_uids=12175693&dopt=Abstract

- **Increased F-18 fluorodeoxyglucose accumulation in a benign neurofibroma--a pitfall in a patient with thyroid cancer: a case report.**
  Author(s): Gabriel M, Erler H, Donnemiller E, Riccabona G.
  Source: Nuklearmedizin. 2002 April; 41(2): N14-5. No Abstract Available.
  http://www.ncbi.nlm.nih.gov:80/entrez/query.fcgi?cmd=Retrieve&db=PubMed&list_uids=11989305&dopt=Abstract

- **Interlaboratory comparison of thyroglobulin measurements for patients with recurrent or metastatic differentiated thyroid cancer.**
  Author(s): Morris LF, Waxman AD, Braunstein GD.
  Source: Clinical Chemistry. 2002 August; 48(8): 1371-2. No Abstract Available.
  http://www.ncbi.nlm.nih.gov:80/entrez/query.fcgi?cmd=Retrieve&db=PubMed&list_uids=12142399&dopt=Abstract

- **Intraepithelial Neutrophils in Thyroid Fine-Needle Aspiration: A Portent of Aggressive Thyroid Cancer?**
  Author(s): Peters SB, Abdelatif O, LiVolsi VA.
  Source: Endocr Pathol. 1996 Spring; 7(1): 47-54.
  http://www.ncbi.nlm.nih.gov:80/entrez/query.fcgi?cmd=Retrieve&db=PubMed&list_uids=12114679&dopt=Abstract

- **Isozyme-specific abnormalities of PKC in thyroid cancer: evidence for post-transcriptional changes in PKC epsilon.**
  Author(s): Knauf JA, Ward LS, Nikiforov YE, Nikiforova M, Puxeddu E, Medvedovic M, Liron T, Mochly-Rosen D, Fagin JA.
  Source: The Journal of Clinical Endocrinology and Metabolism. 2002 May; 87(5): 2150-9.
  http://www.ncbi.nlm.nih.gov:80/entrez/query.fcgi?cmd=Retrieve&db=PubMed&list_uids=11994357&dopt=Abstract

- **Lifestyle and other risk factors for thyroid cancer in Los Angeles County females.**
  Author(s): Mack WJ, Preston-Martin S, Bernstein L, Qian D.

Source: Annals of Epidemiology. 2002 August; 12(6): 395-401.
http://www.ncbi.nlm.nih.gov:80/entrez/query.fcgi?cmd=Retrieve&db=
PubMed&list_uids=12160598&dopt=Abstract

- **Low-iodine diet in the treatment of differentiated thyroid cancer with radioactive iodine.**
  Author(s): Sonenberg M.
  Source: Endocrine. 2002 March; 17(2): 141-3. No Abstract Available.
  http://www.ncbi.nlm.nih.gov:80/entrez/query.fcgi?cmd=Retrieve&db=
  PubMed&list_uids=12041916&dopt=Abstract

- **Management of low-risk well-differentiated thyroid cancer based only on thyroglobulin measurement after recombinant human thyrotropin.**
  Author(s): Wartofsky L.
  Source: Thyroid : Official Journal of the American Thyroid Association. 2002 July; 12(7): 583-90.
  http://www.ncbi.nlm.nih.gov:80/entrez/query.fcgi?cmd=Retrieve&db=
  PubMed&list_uids=12193302&dopt=Abstract

- **Management of papillary and follicular thyroid cancer.**
  Author(s): Jones MK.
  Source: Journal of the Royal Society of Medicine. 2002 July; 95(7): 325-6. No Abstract Available.
  http://www.ncbi.nlm.nih.gov:80/entrez/query.fcgi?cmd=Retrieve&db=
  PubMed&list_uids=12091503&dopt=Abstract

- **Management of thyroid cancer.**
  Author(s): Vini L, Harmer C.
  Source: The Lancet Oncology. 2002 July; 3(7): 407-14. Review.
  http://www.ncbi.nlm.nih.gov:80/entrez/query.fcgi?cmd=Retrieve&db=
  PubMed&list_uids=12142170&dopt=Abstract

- **Managing differentiated thyroid cancer.**
  Author(s): Kendall-Taylor P.
  Source: Bmj (Clinical Research Ed.). 2002 April 27; 324(7344): 988-9. No Abstract Available.
  http://www.ncbi.nlm.nih.gov:80/entrez/query.fcgi?cmd=Retrieve&db=
  PubMed&list_uids=11976226&dopt=Abstract

- **Markov Model-based Estimation of Individual Survival Probability for Medullary Thyroid Cancer Patients.**

Author(s): Esik O, Tusnady G, Tron L, Boer A, Szentirmay Z, Szabolcs I, Racz K, Lengyel E, Szekely J, Kasler M.
Source: Pathology Oncology Research : Por. 2002; 8(2): 93-104.
http://www.ncbi.nlm.nih.gov:80/entrez/query.fcgi?cmd=Retrieve&db=PubMed&list_uids=12172572&dopt=Abstract

- **Matrix metalloproteinases, tissue inhibitors of matrix metalloproteinases and angiogenic cytokines in peripheral blood of patients with thyroid cancer.**
  Author(s): Komorowski J, Pasieka Z, Jankiewicz-Wika J, Stepien H.
  Source: Thyroid : Official Journal of the American Thyroid Association. 2002 August; 12(8): 655-62.
  http://www.ncbi.nlm.nih.gov:80/entrez/query.fcgi?cmd=Retrieve&db=PubMed&list_uids=12225633&dopt=Abstract

- **Mechanisms of aneuploidy in thyroid cancer cell lines and tissues: evidence for mitotic checkpoint dysfunction without mutations in BUB1 and BUBR1.**
  Author(s): Ouyang B, Knauf JA, Ain K, Nacev B, Fagin JA.
  Source: Clinical Endocrinology. 2002 March; 56(3): 341-50.
  http://www.ncbi.nlm.nih.gov:80/entrez/query.fcgi?cmd=Retrieve&db=PubMed&list_uids=11940046&dopt=Abstract

- **Medullary thyroid cancer.**
  Author(s): Kebebew E, Clark OH.
  Source: Curr Treat Options Oncol. 2000 October; 1(4): 359-67. Review.
  http://www.ncbi.nlm.nih.gov:80/entrez/query.fcgi?cmd=Retrieve&db=PubMed&list_uids=12057161&dopt=Abstract

- **Metastatic thyroid cancer visualized on technetium pertechnetate and iodine-131 scintigraphy.**
  Author(s): Verma N, Singh-Wadhwa S, Arvela OM.
  Source: Clinical Nuclear Medicine. 2002 August; 27(8): 610. No Abstract Available.
  http://www.ncbi.nlm.nih.gov:80/entrez/query.fcgi?cmd=Retrieve&db=PubMed&list_uids=12170017&dopt=Abstract

- **Metastin receptor is overexpressed in papillary thyroid cancer and activates MAP kinase in thyroid cancer cells.**
  Author(s): Ringel MD, Hardy E, Bernet VJ, Burch HB, Schuppert F, Burman KD, Saji M.

Source: The Journal of Clinical Endocrinology and Metabolism. 2002 May; 87(5): 2399.
http://www.ncbi.nlm.nih.gov:80/entrez/query.fcgi?cmd=Retrieve&db=PubMed&list_uids=11994395&dopt=Abstract

- **Molecular rearrangements and morphology in thyroid cancer.**
  Author(s): Kroll TG.
  Source: American Journal of Pathology. 2002 June; 160(6): 1941-4. Review. No Abstract Available.
  http://www.ncbi.nlm.nih.gov:80/entrez/query.fcgi?cmd=Retrieve&db=PubMed&list_uids=12057897&dopt=Abstract

- **Multifactorial analysis of survival and recurrences in differentiated thyroid cancer. Comparative evaluation of usefulness of AGES, MACIS, and risk group scores in Mexican population.**
  Author(s): Rodriguez-Cuevas S, Labastida-Almendaro S, Cortes-Arroyo H, Lopez-Garza J, Barroso-Bravo S.
  Source: J Exp Clin Cancer Res. 2002 March; 21(1): 79-86.
  http://www.ncbi.nlm.nih.gov:80/entrez/query.fcgi?cmd=Retrieve&db=PubMed&list_uids=12071534&dopt=Abstract

- **Multinucleated giant cells in fine needle aspirates. Can they help differentiate papillary thyroid cancer from benign nodular goiter?**
  Author(s): Tsou PL, Hsiao YL, Chang TC.
  Source: Acta Cytol. 2002 September-October; 46(5): 823-7.
  http://www.ncbi.nlm.nih.gov:80/entrez/query.fcgi?cmd=Retrieve&db=PubMed&list_uids=12365214&dopt=Abstract

- **Multiple neoplasms in an irradiated cohort: pattern of occurrence and relationship to thyroid cancer outcome.**
  Author(s): Mihailescu D, Shore-Freedman E, Mukani S, Lubin J, Ron E, Schneider AB.
  Source: The Journal of Clinical Endocrinology and Metabolism. 2002 July; 87(7): 3236-41.
  http://www.ncbi.nlm.nih.gov:80/entrez/query.fcgi?cmd=Retrieve&db=PubMed&list_uids=12107231&dopt=Abstract

- **Non-medical exposure to radioiodines and thyroid cancer.**
  Author(s): Hindie E, Leenhardt L, Vitaux F, Colas-Linhart N, Grosclaude P, Galle P, Aurengo A, Bok B.

Source: European Journal of Nuclear Medicine and Molecular Imaging. 2002 August; 29(Supplement 2): S497-512.
http://www.ncbi.nlm.nih.gov:80/entrez/query.fcgi?cmd=Retrieve&db=PubMed&list_uids=12192552&dopt=Abstract

- **Obstructive endotracheal lesions of thyroid cancer.**
  Author(s): Ahmed M, Saleem M, Al-Arifi A, Almahfouz A, Mahasin Z, Al-Sobhi S, Ingemansson S, Taibah K.
  Source: The Journal of Laryngology and Otology. 2002 August; 116(8): 613-21.
  http://www.ncbi.nlm.nih.gov:80/entrez/query.fcgi?cmd=Retrieve&db=PubMed&list_uids=12389690&dopt=Abstract

- **Occupational thyroid cancer?**
  Author(s): Morton WE.
  Source: Journal of Occupational and Environmental Medicine / American College of Occupational and Environmental Medicine. 2002 April; 44(4): 307; Discussion 307-8. No Abstract Available.
  http://www.ncbi.nlm.nih.gov:80/entrez/query.fcgi?cmd=Retrieve&db=PubMed&list_uids=11977414&dopt=Abstract

- **Outcome and toxicity associated with maximum safe dose radioiodine treatment of metastatic thyroid cancer.**
  Author(s): Robeson WR, Ellwood JE, Margulies P, Margouleff D.
  Source: Clinical Nuclear Medicine. 2002 August; 27(8): 556-66.
  http://www.ncbi.nlm.nih.gov:80/entrez/query.fcgi?cmd=Retrieve&db=PubMed&list_uids=12170000&dopt=Abstract

- **Papillary thyroid cancer.**
  Author(s): Yim JH, Doherty GM.
  Source: Curr Treat Options Oncol. 2000 October; 1(4): 329-38. Review.
  http://www.ncbi.nlm.nih.gov:80/entrez/query.fcgi?cmd=Retrieve&db=PubMed&list_uids=12057158&dopt=Abstract

- **Perspective: lessons learned from molecular genetic studies of thyroid cancer--insights into pathogenesis and tumor-specific therapeutic targets.**
  Author(s): Fagin JA.
  Source: Endocrinology. 2002 June; 143(6): 2025-8. No Abstract Available.
  http://www.ncbi.nlm.nih.gov:80/entrez/query.fcgi?cmd=Retrieve&db=PubMed&list_uids=12021165&dopt=Abstract

- **Positron emission tomography in thyroid cancer management.**
  Author(s): Larson SM, Robbins R.
  Source: Semin Roentgenol. 2002 April; 37(2): 169-74.
  http://www.ncbi.nlm.nih.gov:80/entrez/query.fcgi?cmd=Retrieve&db=PubMed&list_uids=12134369&dopt=Abstract

- **Preparation for radioactive iodine administration in differentiated thyroid cancer patients.**
  Author(s): Liel Y.
  Source: Clinical Endocrinology. 2002 October; 57(4): 523-7.
  http://www.ncbi.nlm.nih.gov:80/entrez/query.fcgi?cmd=Retrieve&db=PubMed&list_uids=12354135&dopt=Abstract

- **Prognostic significance of magnetic resonance findings in advanced papillary thyroid cancer.**
  Author(s): Takashima S, Matsushita T, Takayama F, Kadoya M, Fujimori M, Kobayashi T.
  Source: Thyroid: Official Journal of the American Thyroid Association. 2001 December; 11(12): 1153-9.
  http://www.ncbi.nlm.nih.gov:80/entrez/query.fcgi?cmd=Retrieve&db=PubMed&list_uids=12186503&dopt=Abstract

- **Recombinant Human TSH Testing for Recurrent Thyroid Cancer: A Re-appraisal.**
  Author(s): Haber S.
  Source: Thyroid: Official Journal of the American Thyroid Association. 2002 July; 12(7): 599-602. No Abstract Available.
  http://www.ncbi.nlm.nih.gov:80/entrez/query.fcgi?cmd=Retrieve&db=PubMed&list_uids=12193304&dopt=Abstract

- **Recombinant thyrotropin for detection of recurrent thyroid cancer.**
  Author(s): Ladenson PW.
  Source: Trans Am Clin Climatol Assoc. 2002; 113: 21-30.
  http://www.ncbi.nlm.nih.gov:80/entrez/query.fcgi?cmd=Retrieve&db=PubMed&list_uids=12053710&dopt=Abstract

- **Recurrent and/or metastatic thyroid cancer: therapeutic options.**
  Author(s): Karavitaki N, Vlassopoulou V, Tzanela M, Tzavara I, Thalassinos N.

Source: Expert Opinion on Pharmacotherapy. 2002 July; 3(7): 939-47.
http://www.ncbi.nlm.nih.gov:80/entrez/query.fcgi?cmd=Retrieve&db=
PubMed&list_uids=12083993&dopt=Abstract

- **Recurrent or persistent thyroid cancer of follicular cell origin.**
  Author(s): Duren M, Duh QY, Siperstein AE, Clark OH.
  Source: Curr Treat Options Oncol. 2000 October; 1(4): 339-43. Review.
  http://www.ncbi.nlm.nih.gov:80/entrez/query.fcgi?cmd=Retrieve&db=
  PubMed&list_uids=12057159&dopt=Abstract

- **Regulatory subunit type I-alpha of protein kinase A (PRKAR1A): a tumor-suppressor gene for sporadic thyroid cancer.**
  Author(s): Sandrini F, Matyakhina L, Sarlis NJ, Kirschner LS, Farmakidis C, Gimm O, Stratakis CA.
  Source: Genes, Chromosomes & Cancer. 2002 October; 35(2): 182-92.
  http://www.ncbi.nlm.nih.gov:80/entrez/query.fcgi?cmd=Retrieve&db=
  PubMed&list_uids=12203783&dopt=Abstract

- **Relation between Ultrasonographic and Histologic Findings of Tracheal Invasion by Differentiated Thyroid Cancer.**
  Author(s): Yamamura N, Fukushima S, Nakao K, Nakahara M, Kurozumi K, Imabun S, Tsujimoto M.
  Source: World Journal of Surgery. 2002 August; 26(8): 1071-3.
  http://www.ncbi.nlm.nih.gov:80/entrez/query.fcgi?cmd=Retrieve&db=
  PubMed&list_uids=12016485&dopt=Abstract

- **RET expression in papillary thyroid cancer from patients irradiated in childhood for benign conditions.**
  Author(s): Collins BJ, Chiappetta G, Schneider AB, Santoro M, Pentimalli F, Fogelfeld L, Gierlowski T, Shore-Freedman E, Jaffe G, Fusco A.
  Source: The Journal of Clinical Endocrinology and Metabolism. 2002 August; 87(8): 3941-6.
  http://www.ncbi.nlm.nih.gov:80/entrez/query.fcgi?cmd=Retrieve&db=
  PubMed&list_uids=12161537&dopt=Abstract

- **RET Proto-Oncogene and Thyroid Cancer.**
  Author(s): Komminoth P.
  Source: Endocr Pathol. 1997 Autumn; 8(3): 235-239.
  http://www.ncbi.nlm.nih.gov:80/entrez/query.fcgi?cmd=Retrieve&db=
  PubMed&list_uids=12114728&dopt=Abstract

- **Right thyroid hemiagenesis associated with papillary thyroid cancer and an ectopic prelaryngeal thyroid: a case report.**
  Author(s): Huang SM, Chen HD, Wen TY, Kun MS.
  Source: J Formos Med Assoc. 2002 May; 101(5): 368-71.
  http://www.ncbi.nlm.nih.gov:80/entrez/query.fcgi?cmd=Retrieve&db=PubMed&list_uids=12101857&dopt=Abstract

- **Safety of completion thyroidectomy following unilateral lobectomy for well-differentiated thyroid cancer.**
  Author(s): Kupferman ME, Mandel SJ, DiDonato L, Wolf P, Weber RS.
  Source: The Laryngoscope. 2002 July; 112(7 Pt 1): 1209-12.
  http://www.ncbi.nlm.nih.gov:80/entrez/query.fcgi?cmd=Retrieve&db=PubMed&list_uids=12169901&dopt=Abstract

- **Scatter irradiation in childhood causes thyroid cancer.**
  Author(s): Cohen AK, Van Der Schaaf AA.
  Source: The Medical Journal of Australia. 2002 June 17; 176(12): 570-1.
  http://www.ncbi.nlm.nih.gov:80/entrez/query.fcgi?cmd=Retrieve&db=PubMed&list_uids=12064952&dopt=Abstract

- **Scintigraphic evaluation of salivary gland dysfunction in patients with thyroid cancer after radioiodine treatment.**
  Author(s): Caglar M, Tuncel M, Alpar R.
  Source: Clinical Nuclear Medicine. 2002 November; 27(11): 767-71.
  http://www.ncbi.nlm.nih.gov:80/entrez/query.fcgi?cmd=Retrieve&db=PubMed&list_uids=12394122&dopt=Abstract

- **Sensitivity of (123)I whole-body scan and thyroglobulin in the detection of metastases or recurrent differentiated thyroid cancer.**
  Author(s): De Geus-Oei LF, Oei HY, Hennemann G, Krenning EP.
  Source: European Journal of Nuclear Medicine and Molecular Imaging. 2002 June; 29(6): 768-74.
  http://www.ncbi.nlm.nih.gov:80/entrez/query.fcgi?cmd=Retrieve&db=PubMed&list_uids=12029550&dopt=Abstract

- **Sentinel lymph node biopsy in staging of differentiated thyroid cancer: a critical review.**
  Author(s): Wiseman S, Hicks W, Chu Q, Rigual N.
  Source: Surgical Oncology. 2002 November; 11(3): 137.
  http://www.ncbi.nlm.nih.gov:80/entrez/query.fcgi?cmd=Retrieve&db=PubMed&list_uids=12356509&dopt=Abstract

- **Silencing of the PTEN tumor-suppressor gene in anaplastic thyroid cancer.**
  Author(s): Frisk T, Foukakis T, Dwight T, Lundberg J, Hoog A, Wallin G, Eng C, Zedenius J, Larsson C.
  Source: Genes, Chromosomes & Cancer. 2002 September; 35(1): 74-80.
  http://www.ncbi.nlm.nih.gov:80/entrez/query.fcgi?cmd=Retrieve&db=PubMed&list_uids=12203792&dopt=Abstract

- **Somatostatins and their role in thyroid cancer.**
  Author(s): England RJ, Atkin SL.
  Source: Clinical Otolaryngology and Allied Sciences. 2002 April; 27(2): 120-3. Review.
  http://www.ncbi.nlm.nih.gov:80/entrez/query.fcgi?cmd=Retrieve&db=PubMed&list_uids=11994118&dopt=Abstract

- **Surgical approach to cervical lymph node metastasis in differentiated thyroid cancer.**
  Author(s): Goss M, D'Amico S, Mobiglia A, Sargiotto A, Deandrea M.
  Source: Tumori. 2002 May-June; 88(3): S47-8.
  http://www.ncbi.nlm.nih.gov:80/entrez/query.fcgi?cmd=Retrieve&db=PubMed&list_uids=12365389&dopt=Abstract

- **Surveillance of TSH-Suppressive Levothyroxine Treatment in Thyroid Cancer Patients: TRH Testing Versus Basal TSH Determination by a Third Generation Assay.**
  Author(s): Gorges R, Saller B, Eising EG, Quadbeck B, Mann K, Bockisch A.
  Source: Experimental and Clinical Endocrinology & Diabetes : Official Journal, German Society of Endocrinology [and] German Diabetes Association. 2002; 110(7): 355-60.
  http://www.ncbi.nlm.nih.gov:80/entrez/query.fcgi?cmd=Retrieve&db=PubMed&list_uids=12397535&dopt=Abstract

- **Testicular dose and fertility in men following I(131) therapy for thyroid cancer.**
  Author(s): Hyer S, Vini L, O'Connell M, Pratt B, Harmer C.
  Source: Clinical Endocrinology. 2002 June; 56(6): 755-8.
  http://www.ncbi.nlm.nih.gov:80/entrez/query.fcgi?cmd=Retrieve&db=PubMed&list_uids=12072044&dopt=Abstract

- **The accuracy of fine-needle aspiration biopsy and frozen section in patients with thyroid cancer.**

Author(s): Lee TI, Yang HJ, Lin SY, Lee MT, Lin HD, Braverman LE, Tang KT.
Source: Thyroid : Official Journal of the American Thyroid Association. 2002 July; 12(7): 619-26.
http://www.ncbi.nlm.nih.gov:80/entrez/query.fcgi?cmd=Retrieve&db=PubMed&list_uids=12193308&dopt=Abstract

- **The cost effectiveness of dual phase 201Tl thyroid scan in detecting thyroid cancer for evaluating thyroid nodules with equivocal fine-needle aspiration results: the preliminary Taiwanese experience.**
  Author(s): Chen YS, Wang WH, Chan T, Sun SS, Kao A.
  Source: Neoplasma. 2002; 49(2): 129-32.
  http://www.ncbi.nlm.nih.gov:80/entrez/query.fcgi?cmd=Retrieve&db=PubMed&list_uids=12088107&dopt=Abstract

- **The management of thyroid cancer in adults: a review of new guidelines.**
  Author(s): Harris PE.
  Source: Clinical Medicine (London, England). 2002 March-April; 2(2): 144-6.
  http://www.ncbi.nlm.nih.gov:80/entrez/query.fcgi?cmd=Retrieve&db=PubMed&list_uids=11991098&dopt=Abstract

- **The mystery of nm23H1 in thyroid cancer.**
  Author(s): Shi Y, Zou M, Farid NR.
  Source: J Endocrinol Invest. 2002 July-August; 25(7): 663-4. No Abstract Available.
  http://www.ncbi.nlm.nih.gov:80/entrez/query.fcgi?cmd=Retrieve&db=PubMed&list_uids=12150345&dopt=Abstract

- **The proportion of thyroid cancers in the Japanese atomic bomb survivors associated with natural background radiation.**
  Author(s): Little MP.
  Source: Journal of Radiological Protection : Official Journal of the Society for Radiological Protection. 2002 September; 22(3): 279-91.
  http://www.ncbi.nlm.nih.gov:80/entrez/query.fcgi?cmd=Retrieve&db=PubMed&list_uids=12375789&dopt=Abstract

- **The role of radiotherapy in the management of elevated calcitonin after surgery for medullary thyroid cancer.**
  Author(s): Fersht N, Vini L, A'Hern R, Harmer C.

Source: Thyroid : Official Journal of the American Thyroid Association. 2001 December; 11(12): 1161-8.
http://www.ncbi.nlm.nih.gov:80/entrez/query.fcgi?cmd=Retrieve&db=PubMed&list_uids=12186504&dopt=Abstract

- **The use of recombinant thyrotropin in the follow-up of patients with differentiated thyroid cancer.**
  Author(s): Basaria M, Graf H, Cooper DS.
  Source: The American Journal of Medicine. 2002 June 15; 112(9): 721-5.
  http://www.ncbi.nlm.nih.gov:80/entrez/query.fcgi?cmd=Retrieve&db=PubMed&list_uids=12079713&dopt=Abstract

- **Thyroid cancer 15 years after Chernobyl.**
  Author(s): Michel LA, Donckier JE.
  Source: Lancet. 2002 June 1; 359(9321): 1947. No Abstract Available.
  http://www.ncbi.nlm.nih.gov:80/entrez/query.fcgi?cmd=Retrieve&db=PubMed&list_uids=12057581&dopt=Abstract

- **Thyroid cancer after X-ray treatment of benign disorders of the cervical spine in adults.**
  Author(s): Damber L, Johansson L, Johansson R, Larsson LG.
  Source: Acta Oncologica (Stockholm, Sweden). 2002; 41(1): 25-8.
  http://www.ncbi.nlm.nih.gov:80/entrez/query.fcgi?cmd=Retrieve&db=PubMed&list_uids=11990513&dopt=Abstract

- **Thyroid cancer in a child born after the Chernobyl disaster.**
  Author(s): Marks S, Girgis R, Couch R.
  Source: The Lancet Oncology. 2002 September; 3(9): 527-8. No Abstract Available.
  http://www.ncbi.nlm.nih.gov:80/entrez/query.fcgi?cmd=Retrieve&db=PubMed&list_uids=12217789&dopt=Abstract

- **Thyroid cancer in children and adolescents.**
  Author(s): Pacini F.
  Source: J Endocrinol Invest. 2002 July-August; 25(7): 572-3. No Abstract Available.
  http://www.ncbi.nlm.nih.gov:80/entrez/query.fcgi?cmd=Retrieve&db=PubMed&list_uids=12150326&dopt=Abstract

Vocabulary Builder

Adenoma: A noncancerous tumor. [NIH]

Adenosine: A nucleoside that is composed of adenine and d-ribose. Adenosine or adenosine derivatives play many important biological roles in addition to being components of DNA and RNA. Adenosine itself is a neurotransmitter. [NIH]

Adenovirus: A group of viruses that cause respiratory tract and eye infections. Adenoviruses used in gene therapy are altered to carry a specific tumor-fighting gene. [NIH]

Agonists: Drugs that trigger an action from a cell or another drug. [NIH]

Analog: In chemistry, a substance that is similar, but not identical, to another. [NIH]

Apoptosis: A normal series of events in a cell that leads to its death. [NIH]

Aspirate: Fluid withdrawn from a lump, often a cyst, or a nipple. [NIH]

Aspiration: Removal of fluid from a lump, often a cyst, with a needle and a syringe. [NIH]

Assay: Determination of the amount of a particular constituent of a mixture, or of the biological or pharmacological potency of a drug. [EU]

Benign: Not cancerous; does not invade nearby tissue or spread to other parts of the body. [NIH]

Bile: A fluid made by the liver and stored in the gallbladder. Bile is excreted into the small intestine where it helps digest fat. [NIH]

Biochemical: Relating to biochemistry; characterized by, produced by, or involving chemical reactions in living organisms. [EU]

Calcitonin: A hormone secreted by the thyroid that lowers blood calcium levels. [NIH]

Calcium: A mineral found in teeth, bones, and other body tissues. [NIH]

Carcinogenesis: The process by which normal cells are transformed into cancer cells. [NIH]

CEA: Carcinoembryonic antigen. A substance that is sometimes found in an increased amount in the blood of people with certain cancers. [NIH]

Cholesterol: The principal sterol of all higher animals, distributed in body tissues, especially the brain and spinal cord, and in animal fats and oils. [NIH]

Chromosomal: Pertaining to chromosomes. [EU]

Chromosome: Part of a cell that contains genetic information. Except for sperm and eggs, all human cells contain 46 chromosomes. [NIH]

Cyclic: Pertaining to or occurring in a cycle or cycles; the term is applied to chemical compounds that contain a ring of atoms in the nucleus. [EU]

Cystine: A covalently linked dimeric nonessential amino acid formed by the oxidation of cysteine. Two molecules of cysteine are joined together by a disulfide bridge to form cystine. [NIH]

Cytokines: A class of substances that are produced by cells of the immune system and can affect the immune response. Cytokines can also be produced in the laboratory by recombinant DNA technology and given to people to affect immune responses. [NIH]

Drosophila: A genus of small, two-winged flies containing approximately 900 described species. These organisms are the most extensively studied of all genera from the standpoint of genetics and cytology. [NIH]

Ectopic: Pertaining to or characterized by ectopia. [EU]

Endocrinology: A subspecialty of internal medicine concerned with the metabolism, physiology, and disorders of the endocrine system. [NIH]

Endogenous: Produced inside an organism or cell. The opposite is external (exogenous) production. [NIH]

Endoscopy: The use of a thin, lighted tube (called an endoscope) to examine the inside of the body. [NIH]

Epidemiological: Relating to, or involving epidemiology. [EU]

Epirubicin: An anticancer drug that belongs to the family of drugs called antitumor antibiotics. [NIH]

Epithelial: Refers to the cells that line the internal and external surfaces of the body. [NIH]

Epithelium: A thin layer of tissue that covers organs, glands, and other structures within the body. [NIH]

Esophageal: Having to do with the esophagus, the muscular tube through which food passes from the throat to the stomach. [NIH]

Exons: Coding regions of messenger RNA included in the genetic transcript which survive the processing of RNA in cell nuclei to become part of a spliced messenger of structural RNA in the cytoplasm. They include joining and diversity exons of immunoglobulin genes. [NIH]

Fibrosis: The growth of fibrous tissue. [NIH]

Fractionation: Dividing the total dose of radiation therapy into several smaller, equal doses delivered over a period of several days. [NIH]

Glucose: Sugar. [NIH]

Glycoprotein: A protein that has sugar molecules attached to it. [NIH]

Goiter: Enlargement of the thyroid gland. [NIH]

Homeostasis: A tendency to stability in the normal body states (internal environment) of the organism. It is achieved by a system of control mechanisms activated by negative feedback; e.g. a high level of carbon dioxide in extracellular fluid triggers increased pulmonary ventilation, which in turn causes a decrease in carbon dioxide concentration. [EU]

Homologous: Corresponding in structure, position, origin, etc., as (a) the feathers of a bird and the scales of a fish, (b) antigen and its specific antibody, (c) allelic chromosomes. [EU]

Hormonal: Pertaining to or of the nature of a hormone. [EU]

Hybridization: The genetic process of crossbreeding to produce a hybrid. Hybrid nucleic acids can be formed by nucleic acid hybridization of DNA and RNA molecules. Protein hybridization allows for hybrid proteins to be formed from polypeptide chains. [NIH]

Induction: The act or process of inducing or causing to occur, especially the production of a specific morphogenetic effect in the developing embryo through the influence of evocators or organizers, or the production of anaesthesia or unconsciousness by use of appropriate agents. [EU]

Interphase: The interval between two successive cell divisions during which the chromosomes are not individually distinguishable and DNA replication occurs. [NIH]

Invasive: 1. having the quality of invasiveness. 2. involving puncture or incision of the skin or insertion of an instrument or foreign material into the body; said of diagnostic techniques. [EU]

Involution: 1. a rolling or turning inward. 2. one of the movements involved in the gastrulation of many animals. 3. a retrograde change of the entire body or in a particular organ, as the retrograde changes in the female genital organs that result in normal size after delivery. 4. the progressive degeneration occurring naturally with advancing age, resulting in shrivelling of organs or tissues. [EU]

Kinetic: Pertaining to or producing motion. [EU]

Lactation: The period of the secretion of milk. [EU]

Laryngoscope: A thin, lighted tube used to examine the larynx (voice box). [NIH]

Lesion: An area of abnormal tissue change. [NIH]

Levothyroxine: Levo isomer of the thyroid hormone thyroxine. It is used for replacement therapy in reduced or absent thyroid function. [NIH]

Localization: The process of determining or marking the location or site of a lesion or disease. May also refer to the process of keeping a lesion or disease in a specific location or site. [NIH]

Mammary: Pertaining to the mamma, or breast. [EU]

Melanoma: A form of skin cancer that arises in melanocytes, the cells that produce pigment. Melanoma usually begins in a mole. [NIH]

Membrane: A very thin layer of tissue that covers a surface. [NIH]

Mesothelioma: A benign (noncancerous) or malignant (cancerous) tumor affecting the lining of the chest or abdomen. Exposure to asbestos particles in the air increases the risk of developing malignant mesothelioma. [NIH]

Metaphase: The second phase of cell division, in which the chromosomes line up across the equatorial plane of the spindle prior to separation. [NIH]

Metastasis: The spread of cancer from one part of the body to another. Tumors formed from cells that have spread are called "secondary tumors" and contain cells that are like those in the original (primary) tumor. The plural is metastases. [NIH]

Metastatic: Having to do with metastasis, which is the spread of cancer from one part of the body to another. [NIH]

Microscopy: The application of microscope magnification to the study of materials that cannot be properly seen by the unaided eye. [NIH]

Molecular: Of, pertaining to, or composed of molecules : a very small mass of matter. [EU]

Morphology: The science of the form and structure of organisms (plants, animals, and other forms of life). [NIH]

Mutagenesis: Process of generating genetic mutations. It may occur spontaneously or be induced by mutagens. [NIH]

Myeloma: Cancer that arises in plasma cells, a type of white blood cell. [NIH]

Necrosis: Refers to the death of living tissues. [NIH]

Neonatal: Pertaining to the first four weeks after birth. [EU]

Neoplasm: A new growth of benign or malignant tissue. [NIH]

Neoplastic: Pertaining to or like a neoplasm (= any new and abnormal growth); pertaining to neoplasia (= the formation of a neoplasm). [EU]

Neural: 1. pertaining to a nerve or to the nerves. 2. situated in the region of the spinal axis, as the neutral arch. [EU]

Neuroendocrine: Having to do with the interactions between the nervous system and the endocrine system. Describes certain cells that release hormones into the blood in response to stimulation of the nervous system. [NIH]

Neutrophil: A type of white blood cell. [NIH]

Oncogene: A gene that normally directs cell growth. If altered, an oncogene can promote or allow the uncontrolled growth of cancer. Alterations can be inherited or caused by an environmental exposure to carcinogens. [NIH]

Otolaryngology: A surgical specialty concerned with the study and treatment of disorders of the ear, nose, and throat. [NIH]

Ovary: Either of the paired glands in the female that produce the female germ cells and secrete some of the female sex hormones. [NIH]

Pancreatic: Having to do with the pancreas. [NIH]

Parathyroid: 1. situated beside the thyroid gland. 2. one of the parathyroid glands. 3. a sterile preparation of the water-soluble principle(s) of the parathyroid glands, ad-ministered parenterally as an antihypocalcaemic, especially in the treatment of acute hypoparathyroidism with tetany. [EU]

Pathologist: A doctor who identifies diseases by studying cells and tissues under a microscope. [NIH]

Phenotype: The outward appearance of the individual. It is the product of interactions between genes and between the genotype and the environment. This includes the killer phenotype, characteristic of YEASTS. [NIH]

Phosphorylation: The introduction of a phosphoryl group into a compound through the formation of an ester bond between the compound and a phosphorus moiety. [NIH]

Prevalence: The total number of cases of a given disease in a specified population at a designated time. It is differentiated from incidence, which refers to the number of new cases in the population at a given time. [NIH]

Progression: Increase in the size of a tumor or spread of cancer in the body. [NIH]

Proteins: Polymers of amino acids linked by peptide bonds. The specific sequence of amino acids determines the shape and function of the protein. [NIH]

PTC: Percutaneous transhepatic cholangiography (per-kyoo-TAN-ee-us trans-heh-PAT-ik ko-LAN-jee-AH-gra-fee). A procedure to x-ray the bile ducts. In this procedure, a dye is injected through a thin needle inserted through the skin into the liver or the gallbladder, and an x-ray picture is taken. [NIH]

Radioisotope: An unstable element that releases radiation as it breaks down. Radioisotopes can be used in imaging tests or as a treatment for cancer. [NIH]

Receptor: A molecule inside or on the surface of a cell that binds to a specific substance and causes a specific physiologic effect in the cell. [NIH]

Recombinant: 1. a cell or an individual with a new combination of genes not found together in either parent; usually applied to linked genes. [EU]

Recurrence: The return of cancer, at the same site as the original (primary) tumor or in another location, after the tumor had disappeared. [NIH]

Registries: The systems and processes involved in the establishment, support, management, and operation of registers, e.g., disease registers. [NIH]

Remission: A decrease in or disappearance of signs and symptoms of cancer. In partial remission, some, but not all, signs and symptoms of cancer have disappeared. In complete remission, all signs and symptoms of cancer have disappeared, although there still may be cancer in the body. [NIH]

Resection: Removal of tissue or part or all of an organ by surgery. [NIH]

Retinoid: Vitamin A or a vitamin A-like compound. [NIH]

Rheumatoid: Resembling rheumatism. [EU]

Secretion: 1. the process of elaborating a specific product as a result of the activity of a gland; this activity may range from separating a specific substance of the blood to the elaboration of a new chemical substance. 2. any substance produced by secretion. [EU]

Serum: The clear liquid part of the blood that remains after blood cells and clotting proteins have been removed. [NIH]

Species: A taxonomic category subordinate to a genus (or subgenus) and superior to a subspecies or variety, composed of individuals possessing common characters distinguishing them from other categories of individuals of the same taxonomic level. In taxonomic nomenclature, species are designated by the genus name followed by a Latin or Latinized adjective or noun. [EU]

Sporadic: Neither endemic nor epidemic; occurring occasionally in a random or isolated manner. [EU]

Stabilization: The creation of a stable state. [EU]

Stomach: An organ that is part of the digestive system. It helps in the digestion of food by mixing it with digestive juices and churning it into a thin liquid. [NIH]

Supplementation: Adding nutrients to the diet. [NIH]

Suppressive: Tending to suppress : effecting suppression; specifically : serving to suppress activity, function, symptoms. [EU]

Technetium: The first artificially produced element and a radioactive fission product of uranium. The stablest isotope has a mass number 99 and is used diagnostically as a radioactive imaging agent. Technetium has the atomic symbol Tc, atomic number 43, and atomic weight 98.91. [NIH]

Telomerase: Essential ribonucleoprotein reverse transcriptase that adds telomeric DNA to the ends of eukaryotic chromosomes. Telomerase appears to be repressed in normal human somatic tissues but reactivated in cancer, and thus may be necessary for malignant transformation. EC 2.7.7.-. [NIH]

Thyrotoxicosis: The condition resulting from presentation to the tissues of excessive quantities of the thyroid hormones, whether the excess results from overproduction by the thyroid gland (as in Graves' disease), originated outside the thyroid, or is due to loss of storage function and leakage from the gland. [EU]

Thyrotropin: A peptide hormone secreted by the anterior pituitary. It promotes the growth of the thyroid gland and stimulates the synthesis of thyroid hormones and the release of thyroxine by the thyroid gland. [NIH]

Topotecan: An anticancer drug that belongs to the family drugs called topoisomerase inhibitors. [NIH]

Toxicity: The quality of being poisonous, especially the degree of virulence of a toxic microbe or of a poison. [EU]

Toxins: Poisons produced by certain animals, plants, or bacteria. [NIH]

Tracer: A substance (such as a radioisotope) used in imaging procedures. [NIH]

Tyrosine: A non-essential amino acid. In animals it is synthesized from phenylalanine. It is also the precursor of epinephrine, thyroid hormones, and melanin. [NIH]

Ultrasonography: A procedure in which sound waves (called ultrasound) are bounced off tissues and the echoes are converted to a picture (sonogram). [NIH]

Withdrawal: 1. a pathological retreat from interpersonal contact and social involvement, as may occur in schizophrenia, depression, or schizoid avoidant and schizotypal personality disorders. 2. (DSM III-R) a substance-specific organic brain syndrome that follows the cessation of use or reduction in intake of a psychoactive substance that had been regularly used to induce a state of intoxication. [EU]

Xenograft: The cells of one species transplanted to another species. [NIH]

CHAPTER 5. BOOKS ON THYROID CANCER

Overview

This chapter provides bibliographic book references relating to thyroid cancer. You have many options to locate books on thyroid cancer. The simplest method is to go to your local bookseller and inquire about titles that they have in stock or can special order for you. Some patients, however, feel uncomfortable approaching their local booksellers and prefer online sources (e.g. **www.amazon.com** and **www.bn.com**). In addition to online booksellers, excellent sources for book titles on thyroid cancer include the Combined Health Information Database and the National Library of Medicine. Once you have found a title that interests you, visit your local public or medical library to see if it is available for loan.

Book Summaries: Federal Agencies

The Combined Health Information Database collects various book abstracts from a variety of healthcare institutions and federal agencies. To access these summaries, go to **http://chid.nih.gov/detail/detail.html**. You will need to use the "Detailed Search" option. To find book summaries, use the drop boxes at the bottom of the search page where "You may refine your search by." Select the dates and language you prefer. For the format option, select "Monograph/Book." Now type "thyroid cancer" (or synonyms) into the "For these words:" box. You will only receive results on books. You should check back periodically with this database which is updated every 3 months. The following is a typical result when searching for books on thyroid cancer:

- **Cancer Incidence in Chinese, Japanese, and Filipinos in the U.S. and Asia, 1988-1992**

    Source: Union City, CA, Northern California Cancer Center, 1999.

    Contact: Northern California Cancer Center, 32960 Alvarado-Niles Road, Suite 600, Union City, CA 94587. (510) 429-2500. INTERNET/EMAIL: http://www.nccc.org.

    Summary: Cancer Incidence in Chinese, Japanese, and Filipinos in the U.S. and Asia, 1988-1992, provides a useful resource of cancer information for Chinese, Japanese, and Filipino populations in the United States and Asia. The intended audience are researchers, health care professionals, and the general public. The authors include descriptions of specific cancers, their risk factors, and their patterns of occurrence to provide the reader with an overview of cancer in these three largest Asian populations in northern California. Data are from cancer registries in China, Hong Kong, Singapore, Japan, the Philippines, and the United States. Cancer incidence and population data are grouped according to geographic location in Asia, and by race/ethnicity in the United States. The authors caution that comparing the data from different regions must be considered in relation to (1) case identification, (2) data collected, (3) quality assurance and data management, and (4) confidentiality. The authors provide specific data for the following cancers: (1) Biliary tract, (2) breast, (3) cervix and uterus, (4) colon, (5) esophagus, (6) liver, (7) lung, (8) nasopharynx, (9) ovary, (10) pancreas, (11) prostate, (12) rectum, (13) stomach, (14) thyroid, (15) bladder, and (16) non-Hodgkin's lymphoma. The authors conclude with several appendixes, including (1) population distributions in Asia and the United States by age and sex, (2) site recodes for incidence data, and (3) data sources.

The National Library of Medicine Book Index

The National Library of Medicine at the National Institutes of Health has a massive database of books published on healthcare and biomedicine. Go to the following Internet site, **http://locatorplus.gov/**, and then select "Search LOCATORplus." Once you are in the search area, simply type "thyroid cancer" (or synonyms) into the search box, and select "books only." From there, results can be sorted by publication date, author, or relevance. The following was recently catalogued by the National Library of Medicine:[31]

---

[31] In addition to LOCATORPlus, in collaboration with authors and publishers, the National Center for Biotechnology Information (NCBI) is adapting biomedical books for the Web. The

- **Bone metastases of thyroid cancer, biological behaviour and therapeutic possibilities.** Author: Jan Nemec ... [et al.]; Year: 1978; Praha: Univerzita Karlova, 1978.

- **Cancer of the thyroid gland [by] Oliver H. Beahrs [and] Bart M. Pasternak.** Author: Beahrs, Oliver Howard, 1914-; Year: 1969; Chicago, Year Book Medical Publishers, 1969.

- **Cancer of the thyroid, by John de J. Pemberton and B. Marden Black.** Author: Pemberton, John de J. (John de Jarnette), 1887-; Year: 1954; [New York] American Cancer Society [c1954]

- **Carcinoma of the thyroid.** Author: edited by Jonas T. Johnson and Jack L. Gluckman; Year: 1999; Oxford: Isis Medical Media; Herndon, Va.: Distributed in the USA by Books International, 1999. ISBN: 1899066853 http://www.amazon.com/exec/obidos/ASIN/1899066853/icongroupinterna

- **Controversies in the management of differentiated thyroid cancer.** Author: edited by B. Cady ... [et al.]; Year: 1987; [Leiden?]: Boerhaave Committee for Postgraduate Medical Education, University of Leiden, [1987] ISBN: 9067671363

- **Estimated exposures and thyroid doses received by the American people from iodine-131 in fallout following Nevada atmospheric nuclear bomb tests microform: a report.** Author: from the National Cancer Institute; Year: 1997; [Washington, D.C.]: U.S. Department of Health and Human Services, National Institutes of Health, National Cancer Institute, [1997]

- **Health provider's guide to contraception. International.** Author: C.W. Porter, Jr., R.S. Waife, H.R. Holtrop; Year: 1983; Chestnut Hill., Pathfinder Fund, 1983.

- **Histogenesis of thyroid cancer.** Author: Simionescu, N. (Nicolae); Year: 1970; London, Heinemann [1970] ISBN: 0433302801

- **Induction of thyroid cancer by ionizing radiation: recommendations of the National Council on Radiation Protection and Measurements.** Author: National Council on Radiation Protection and Measurements; Year: 1985; Bethesda, Md.: The Council, c1985. ISBN: 0913392723

---

books may be accessed in two ways: (1) by searching directly using any search term or phrase (in the same way as the bibliographic database PubMed), or (2) by following the links to PubMed abstracts. Each PubMed abstract has a "Books" button that displays a facsimile of the abstract in which some phrases are hypertext links. These phrases are also found in the books available at NCBI. Click on hyperlinked results in the list of books in which the phrase is found. Currently, the majority of the links are between the books and PubMed. In the future, more links will be created between the books and other types of information, such as gene and protein sequences and macromolecular structures. See **http://www.ncbi.nlm.nih.gov/entrez/query.fcgi?db=Books.**

http://www.amazon.com/exec/obidos/ASIN/0913392723/icongroupinterna

- **Irradiation-related thyroid cancer: information for physicians.** Author: prepared by the Division of Cancer Control and Rehabilitation, National Cancer Institute; Year: 1977; [Bethesda, Md.]: U. S. Dept. of Health, Education, and Welfare, Public Health Service, National Institutes of Health, [1977?]
- **Oversight on implementation of the Orphan Drug Act (Public Law 97-414): hearing before the Committee on Labor and Human Resources, United States Senate, Ninety-eighth Congress, first session, on reviewing the radioepidemiological tables and thyroid cance.** Author: United States. Congress. Senate. Committee on Labor and Human Resources; Year: 1984; Washington: U.S. G.P.O., 1984.
- **Radiation and thyroid cancer.** Author: editors, G. Thomas, A. Karaoglou, E.D. Williams; Year: 1999; Singapore; River Edge, NJ: World Scientific, c1999. ISBN: 9810238142
  http://www.amazon.com/exec/obidos/ASIN/9810238142/icongroupinterna
- **Report of the Expert Meeting on Thyroid Cancer After the Chernobyl Accident: Kiev, Ukraine, 18-21 October 1993.** Author: World Health Organization, International Programme on Health Effects of the Chernobyl Accident (IPHECA); Year: 1994; Geneva: World Health Organization, 1994.
- **Scientific protocol for the study of thyroid cancer and other thyroid disease in Belarus following the Chernobyl accident.** Author: prepared by U.S. committee, David V. Becker, chaiman ... [et al.]; Year: 1992; [United States: s.n., 1992?]
- **Soft tissue roentogenography in diagnosis of thyroid cancer; detection of psammoma bodies by spot-tangential projection, by Masayoshi Akisada and Yoshihide Fujimoto.** Author: Akisada, Masayoshi; Year: 1973; Tokyo, Igaku Shoin, 1973.
- **Thyroglobulin and thyroglobulin antibodies in the follow-up of thyroid cancer and endemic goiter: workshop proceeding Schilddrüse 1985.** Author: edited by Michael Hüfner and Christoph Reiners; Year: 1987; Stuttgart; New York: Thieme, 1987. ISBN: 3136981014
- **Thyroid and parathyroid disorders: 1998 Cherry Blossom Conference.** Author: Maisie L. Shindo and Gregory W. Randolph, editors; Year: 2002; Alexandria, VA: American Academy of Otolaryngology--Head and Neck Surgery Foundation, 2002. ISBN: 1567720420
  http://www.amazon.com/exec/obidos/ASIN/1567720420/icongroupinterna

- **Thyroid cancer: a comprehensive guide to clinical management.** Author: edited by Leonard Wartofsky; foreword by Ernest L. Mazzaferri; Year: 2000; Totowa, N.J.: Humana Press, c2000. ISBN: 0896034291
  http://www.amazon.com/exec/obidos/ASIN/0896034291/icongroupinterna

- **Thyroid cancer: a report by 76 Illinois hospitals on patients diagnosed in 1970-84.** Author: Expert Meeting on Thyroid Cancer After the Chernobyl Accident (1993: Kiev, Ukraine); Year: 1990; Chicago (77 E. Monroe St., Chicago 60603): American Cancer Society, Illinois Division, c1990.

- **Thyroid cancer: diagnosis and treatment.** Author: edited by Orlo H. Clark, Shiro Noguchi; cover illustration by Emilie Clark; Year: 2000; St. Louis, Mo.: Quality Medical Pub., 2000. ISBN: 1576261166
  http://www.amazon.com/exec/obidos/ASIN/1576261166/icongroupinterna

- **Thyroid cancer: its epidemiology, clinical features, and treatment.** Author: Georg Riccabona; Year: 1987; Berlin; New York: Springer-Verlag, c1987. ISBN: 038716555X
  http://www.amazon.com/exec/obidos/ASIN/038716555X/icongroupinterna

- **Thyroid cancer: proceedings of the First European Symposium on Thyroid Cancer, Montpellier, 6-7 June 1985.** Author: editors, C. Jaffiol and G. Milhaud; Year: 1985; Amsterdam; New York: Excerpta Medica; New York, NY, USA: Sole distributors for the USA and Canada, Elsevier Science Pub. Co., 1985. ISBN: 0444807594
  http://www.amazon.com/exec/obidos/ASIN/0444807594/icongroupinterna

- **Thyroid cancer: role of radionuclides in diagnosis, management, and treatment: proceedings of the National Seminar on Thyroid Cancer: Role of Radionuclides in Diagnosis, Management, and Treatment.** Author: sponsored by World Health Organizationand Bhabha Atomic; Year: 1986; Bombay, India: Radiation Medicine Centre, Bhabha Atomic Research Centre, c1986.

- **Thyroid cancer in Denmark in the period 1943-1968.** Author: by Finn Lindahl; Year: 1976; Copenhagen: FADL's Forlag, 1976. ISBN: 8774375717
  http://www.amazon.com/exec/obidos/ASIN/8774375717/icongroupinterna

- **Thyroid cancer.** Author: 3rd International Thyroid Symposium, Univ.-Klinik für Nuklearmedizin, Innsbruck, Austria, September 13-15, 1982; president, Georg Riccabona, co-president, O. Dapunt; organizing committee, H. Fill ... [et al.]; Year: 1983; Copenhagen: [s.n.], 1983. ISBN: 8774942484

- **Thyroid cancer.** Author: edited by William Duncan; Year: 1980; Berlin; New York: Springer-Verlag, 1980. ISBN: 3540093281

- **Thyroid cancer.** Author: editor, Larry D. Greenfield; Year: 1978; Cleveland: CRC Press, c1978. ISBN: 0849352053
  http://www.amazon.com/exec/obidos/ASIN/0849352053/icongroupinterna

- **Thyroid cancer.** Author: edited by James A. Fagin; Year: 1998; Boston: Kluwer Academic, c1998. ISBN: 0792383265
  http://www.amazon.com/exec/obidos/ASIN/0792383265/icongroupinterna

- **Thyroid cancer.** Author: H.-J. Biersack, F. Grünwald (eds.); Year: 2001; Berlin; New York: Springer, c2001. ISBN: 3540413901
  http://www.amazon.com/exec/obidos/ASIN/3540413901/icongroupinterna

- **Treatment of thyroid cancer in childhood: proceedings of a workshop held September 10-11, 1992 at the National Institutes of Health, in Bethesda, Maryland.** Author: edited by Jacob Robbins; Year: 1994; [Bethesda, Md.: National Institutes of Health]; Springfield, VA: Available from the US Dept. of Commerce, Technology Administration, National Technical Information Service, [1994]

Chapters on Thyroid Cancer

Frequently, thyroid cancer will be discussed within a book, perhaps within a specific chapter. In order to find chapters that are specifically dealing with thyroid cancer, an excellent source of abstracts is the Combined Health Information Database. You will need to limit your search to book chapters and thyroid cancer using the "Detailed Search" option. Go directly to the following hyperlink: **http://chid.nih.gov/detail/detail.html**. To find book chapters, use the drop boxes at the bottom of the search page where "You may refine your search by." Select the dates and language you prefer, and the format option "Book Chapter." By making these selections and typing in "thyroid cancer" (or synonyms) into the "For these words:" box, you will only receive results on chapters in books. The following is a typical result when searching for book chapters on thyroid cancer:

- **Endocrine Disease**

    Source: in Miller, R.L., et al. General and Oral Pathology for the Dental Hygienist. St. Louis, MO: Mosby-Year Book, Inc. 1995. p. 309-320.

    Contact: Available from Mosby-Year Book, Inc. 11830 Westline Industrial Drive, St. Louis, MO 63146-9934. (800) 426-4545 or (314) 872-8370; Fax (800) 535-9935 or (314) 432-1380; E-mail: customer.support@mosby.com; http://www.mosby.com. Price: $43.00 plus shipping and handling. ISBN: 0801670241. Stock Number 07024.

    Summary: This chapter, from a textbook on pathology for dental hygiene students, covers endocrine disease. Topics include the clinical aspects of hyper-and hypopituitarism; diabetes insipidus; the development of the thyroid gland, and the physiology and function of the thyroglossal duct cyst and the lingual thyroid gland; common causes of myxedema; the etiology of Hashimoto's disease; the etiology and clinical symptoms of Graves' disease; thyroid cancer and its relationship to radiation or genetic etiology; goiter; the etiology, pathogenesis, and clinical features of Friderichsen-Waterhouse syndrome, Addison's disease, and Cushing's syndrome; diseases caused by hypersecretion of aldosterone and adrenal sex hormones; the clinical and radiographic changes indicative of hyperparathyroidism; diabetes mellitus (types I and II); and common dental problems associated with diabetes mellitus. The chapter includes a list of learning objectives; illustrative case studies; and recommended readings. 4 figures. 2 tables.

General Home References

In addition to references for thyroid cancer, you may want a general home medical guide that spans all aspects of home healthcare. The following list is a recent sample of such guides (sorted alphabetically by title; hyperlinks provide rankings, information, and reviews at Amazon.com):

- **Cancer: 50 Essential Things to Do** by Greg Anderson, O. Carl Simonton; Paperback - 184 pages; Revised & Updated edition (August 1999), Plume; ISBN: 0452280745;

    http://www.amazon.com/exec/obidos/ASIN/0452280745/icongroupinterna

- **Cancer Encyclopedia -- Collections of Anti-Cancer & Anti-Carcinogenic Agents, Chemicals, Drugs and Substances** by John C. Bartone; Paperback (January 2002), ABBE Publishers Association of Washington, DC; ISBN: 0788326791;

    http://www.amazon.com/exec/obidos/ASIN/0788326791/icongroupinterna

- **Cancer Sourcebook: Basic Consumer Health Information About Major Forms and Stages of Cancer** by Edward J. Prucha (Editor); Library Binding - 1100 pages, 3rd edition (August 1, 2000), Omnigraphics, Inc.; ISBN: 0780802276;
  http://www.amazon.com/exec/obidos/ASIN/0780802276/icongroupinterna

- **Cancer Supportive Care: A Comprehensive Guide for Patients and Their Families** by Ernest H. Rosenbaum, M.D., Isadora Rosenbaum, M.A.; Paperback - 472 pages (November 5, 1998), Somerville House Books Limited; ISBN: 1894042115;
  http://www.amazon.com/exec/obidos/ASIN/1894042115/icongroupinterna

- **Cancer Symptom Management: Patient Self-Care Guides (Book with CD-ROM for Windows & Macintosh)** by Connie Henke Yarbro (Editor), et al; CD-ROM - 264 pages, 2nd Book & CD-Rom edition (January 15, 2000), Jones & Bartlett Publishing; ISBN: 0763711675;
  http://www.amazon.com/exec/obidos/ASIN/0763711675/icongroupinterna

- **Diagnosis Cancer: Your Guide Through the First Few Months** by Wendy Schlessel Harpham, Ann Bliss Pilcher (Illustrator); Paperback: 230 pages; Revised & Updated edition (November 1997), .W. Norton & Company; ISBN: 0393316912;
  http://www.amazon.com/exec/obidos/ASIN/0393316912/icongroupinterna

- **The Human Side of Cancer: Living with Hope, Coping with Uncertainty** by Jimmie C. Holland, M.D., Sheldon Lewis; Paperback - 368 pages (October 2, 2001), Quill; ISBN: 006093042X;
  http://www.amazon.com/exec/obidos/ASIN/006093042X/icongroupinterna

Vocabulary Builder

Biliary: Having to do with the liver, bile ducts, and/or gallbladder. [NIH]

Bladder: The organ that stores urine. [NIH]

Carcinogenic: Producing carcinoma. [EU]

Cervix: The lower, narrow end of the uterus that forms a canal between the uterus and vagina. [NIH]

Contraception: The prevention of conception or impregnation. [EU]

Endemic: Present or usually prevalent in a population or geographical area at all times; said of a disease or agent. Called also endemial. [EU]

Endometrium: The layer of tissue that lines the uterus. [NIH]

Esophagus: The muscular tube through which food passes from the throat to the stomach. [NIH]

Hypersecretion: Excessive secretion. [EU]

Indicative: That indicates; that points out more or less exactly; that reveals fairly clearly. [EU]

Larynx: The area of the throat containing the vocal cords and used for breathing, swallowing, and talking. Also called the voice box. [NIH]

Myxedema: A condition characterized by a dry, waxy type of swelling with abnormal deposits of mucin in the skin and other tissues. It is produced by a functional insufficiency of the thyroid gland, resulting in deficiency of thyroid hormone. The skin becomes puffy around the eyes and on the cheeks and the face is dull and expressionless with thickened nose and lips. The congenital form of the disease is cretinism. [NIH]

Nasopharynx: The upper part of the throat behind the nose. An opening on each side of the nasopharynx leads into the ear. [NIH]

Oral: By or having to do with the mouth. [NIH]

Pancreas: A glandular organ located in the abdomen. It makes pancreatic juices, which contain enzymes that aid in digestion, and it produces several hormones, including insulin. The pancreas is surrounded by the stomach, intestines, and other organs. [NIH]

Rectum: The last 8 to 10 inches of the large intestine. [NIH]

Testis: Either of the paired male reproductive glands that produce the male germ cells and the male hormones. [NIH]

Uterus: The small, hollow, pear-shaped organ in a woman's pelvis. This is the organ in which a fetus develops. Also called the womb. [NIH]

CHAPTER 6. MULTIMEDIA ON THYROID CANCER

Overview

Information on thyroid cancer can come in a variety of formats. Among multimedia sources, video productions, slides, audiotapes, and computer databases are often available. In this chapter, we show you how to keep current on multimedia sources of information on thyroid cancer. We start with sources that have been summarized by federal agencies, and then show you how to find bibliographic information catalogued by the National Library of Medicine. If you see an interesting item, visit your local medical library to check on the availability of the title.

Bibliography: Multimedia on Thyroid Cancer

The National Library of Medicine is a rich source of information on healthcare-related multimedia productions including slides, computer software, and databases. To access the multimedia database, go to the following Web site: **http://locatorplus.gov/**. Select "Search LOCATORplus." Once in the search area, simply type in thyroid cancer (or synonyms). Then, in the option box provided below the search box, select "Audiovisuals and Computer Files." From there, you can choose to sort results by publication date, author, or relevance. The following multimedia has been indexed on thyroid cancer. For more information, follow the hyperlink indicated:

- **Anterior neck: the thyroid area.** Source: Veterans Administration Dental Training Center; Year: 1969; Format: Motion picture; Washington: The Center; [Atlanta: for loan by National Medical Audiovisual Center, 1969]

- **Cancer of the thyroid gland : treatment of a case by radio-active iodine.** Source: [produced by the American Medical Association]; Year: 1947; Format: Motion picture; United States: [s.n.], 1947.
- **Cancer of the thyroid, salivary glands, and other head and neck sites.** Source: American College of Surgeons; Year: 1979; Format: Sound recording; Chicago: The College, 1979.
- **Controversies in thyroid cancer therapy, adrenal imaging and osteoporosis evaluation.** Source: the Society of Nuclear Medicine; Year: 1992; Format: Slide; [New York, NY]: The Society, [1992]
- **Current management of thyroid cancer.** Source: SSO, the Society of Surgical Oncology, 52nd Annual Cancer Symposium, March 4-7, 1999, Orlando, FL; Year: 1999; Format: Videorecording; [Chicago, Ill.]: Distributed by Teach'em, [1999]
- **Dissection of the parathyroid and thyroid glands.** Source: Montefiore Hospital and Medical Center; Year: 1970; Format: Motion picture; Bronx, [N. Y.]: The Center, [1970]
- **Focus: your thyroid patient.** Source: Herbert A. Selenkow; produced by Robert P. Goldman; Year: 1975; Format: Motion picture; Elkhart, Ind.: Ames Co., 1975.
- **From head to toe.** Source: Abbot Laboratories; [made by] Gilbert Altschul Productions, inc; Year: 1968; Format: Motion picture; [North Chicago]: The Laboratories, 1968.
- **In vitro thyroid studies.** Source: Nuclear Associates; produced by Medical Multimedia Corp; Year: 1974; Format: Slide; New York: Nuclear Associates, c1974.
- **Major endocrine disorders: thyroid.** Source: Univ. of California, San Francisco Medical Center, Continuing Education in the Health Sciences; Year: 1968; Format: Motion picture; San Francisco: Univ. of Calif., Educational TV Div., [1968]
- **Management of a thyroid nodule.** Source: Penn State Television, WPSX-TV; Year: 1978; Format: Videorecording; University Park, Pa.: Pennsylvania State Univ.: [for loan and sale by its Audio-Visual Services], c1978.
- **Neoplasms of the thyroid gland.** Source: Educational Research and Development Laboratory, School of Medicine, University of Missouri; Year: 1969; Format: Slide; Columbia: The School: [for sale by Univ. of Missouri-Columbia, Medical Center, Educational Resources Group], 1969.
- **Papillary adenocarcinoma of the thyroid gland.** Source: Mayo Clinic; Year: 1956; Format: Motion picture; Rochester, Minn.: The Clinic, 1956.

- **Pitfalls in thyroid diagnosis.** Source: with Norman Rosenthal; Year: 1990; Format: Videorecording; Secaucus, N.J.: Network for Continuing Medical Education, c1990.
- **Radical neck dissection for carcinoma of the thyroid.** Source: U. S. Naval Hospital, St. Albans, New York; Year: 1955; Format: Motion picture; St. Albans, N. Y.: The Hospital; [Bethesda, Md.: for loan by National Naval Medical Center Audiovisual Resources Division:, 1955]
- **Radioisotopes : their application to humans as tracer studies and for therapeutic use.** Source: Medical Film Guild, Ltd; Year: 1953; Format: Motion picture; United States: The Guild, [1953]
- **Surgical management of thyroid cancer-total thyroidectomy.** Source: American College of Surgeons; produced and distributed by DG, Davis & Geck; Year: 1983; Format: Videorecording; Danbury, Conn.: American Cyanamid, c1983.
- **Thyroid and bone cancer.** Source: University of Texas, System Cancer Center, M. D. Anderson Hospital and Tumor Institute; [produced by] MDA-TV; Year: 1974; Format: Videorecording; Houston: The Center, 1974.
- **Thyroid cancer .** Year: 1992; Format: Slide; [Columbus, Ohio]: Ohio Medical Education Network, [1992]
- **Thyroid cancer: diagnosis and treatment.** Source: American Cancer Society, inc.; [made by] Aegis Productions, inc; Year: 1969; Format: Motion picture; [New York]: The Society, 1969.
- **Thyroid cancer.** Source: Department of Continuing Medical Education School of Medicine State University of New York at Buffalo, in cooperation with the Lakes Area Regional Medical Program; Year: 1975; Format: Slide; [Buffalo]: Communications in Learning, 1975.
- **Thyroid disease as a late sequela of radioactive fallout.** Source: Austin Lowrey; produced by Robert Strovink; Year: 1971; Format: Motion picture; Morton Grove, Ill.: Flint Laboratories, [1971]
- **Thyroid diseases: diagnosis and treatment.** Source: Trainex Corporation; Year: 1975; Format: Filmstrip; Garden Grove, Calif.: Trainex, c1975.
- **Thyroid physiology and disease : thyroid nodules and cancer.** Source: a National Medical Audiovisual Center production; [presented by] the U.S. Department of Health, Education, and Welfare, Public Health Service; Year: 1969; Format: Motion picture; United States: The Service, 1969.
- **Thyroid today: an endocrine update.** Source: Flint Laboratories; produced by Medcom, Inc; Year: 1973; Format: Motion picture; Deerfield, Ill.: The Laboratories, [1973]

- **Thyroid.** Source: [presented by the Ohio Medical Education Network]; Year: 1988; Format: Slide; [Columbus, Ohio]: The Network, [1988]
- **Thyroidectomy.** Source: author, Orlo H. Clark; produced by DG, Davis & Geck; Year: 1986; Format: Videorecording; Danbury, Conn.: American Cyanamid, c1986.
- **Total en bloc spondylectomy by posterior approach.** Source: American Academy of Orthopaedic Surgeons; Kanazawa University, Department of Orthopaedic Surgery; Year: 1995; Format: Videorecording; [Rosemont, Ill.]: The Academy, c1995.
- **Total thyroidectomy for c-cell hyperplasia or medullary carcinoma.** Source: produced by Ciné-Med; Year: 1992; Format: Videorecording; [Wayne, N.J.]: American Cyanamid, c1992.
- **Understanding thyroid function testing.** Source: University of Michigan Medical Center; Year: 1973; Format: Slide; [Ann Arbor, Mich.]: The University, [1970?]

Vocabulary Builder

Adenocarcinoma: Cancer that begins in cells that line certain internal organs and that have glandular (secretory) properties. [NIH]

Hyperplasia: An abnormal increase in the number of cells in an organ or tissue. [NIH]

Orthopaedic: Pertaining to the correction of deformities of the musculoskeletal system; pertaining to orthopaedics. [EU]

Osteoporosis: A condition that is characterized by a decrease in bone mass and density, causing bones to become fragile. [NIH]

Posterior: Situated in back of, or in the back part of, or affecting the back or dorsal surface of the body. In lower animals, it refers to the caudal end of the body. [EU]

Sequela: Any lesion or affection following or caused by an attack of disease. [EU]

CHAPTER 7. PERIODICALS AND NEWS ON THYROID CANCER

Overview

Keeping up on the news relating to thyroid cancer can be challenging. Subscribing to targeted periodicals can be an effective way to stay abreast of recent developments on thyroid cancer. Periodicals include newsletters, magazines, and academic journals.

In this chapter, we suggest a number of news sources and present various periodicals that cover thyroid cancer beyond and including those which are published by patient associations mentioned earlier. We will first focus on news services, and then on periodicals. News services, press releases, and newsletters generally use more accessible language, so if you do chose to subscribe to one of the more technical periodicals, make sure that it uses language you can easily follow.

News Services & Press Releases

Well before articles show up in newsletters or the popular press, they may appear in the form of a press release or a public relations announcement. One of the simplest ways of tracking press releases on thyroid cancer is to search the news wires. News wires are used by professional journalists, and have existed since the invention of the telegraph. Today, there are several major "wires" that are used by companies, universities, and other organizations to announce new medical breakthroughs. In the following sample of sources, we will briefly describe how to access each service. These services only post recent news intended for public viewing.

PR Newswire

Perhaps the broadest of the wires is PR Newswire Association, Inc. To access this archive, simply go to **http://www.prnewswire.com**. Below the search box, select the option "The last 30 days." In the search box, type "thyroid cancer" or synonyms. The search results are shown by order of relevance. When reading these press releases, do not forget that the sponsor of the release may be a company or organization that is trying to sell a particular product or therapy. Their views, therefore, may be biased.

Reuters

The Reuters' Medical News database can be very useful in exploring news archives relating to thyroid cancer. While some of the listed articles are free to view, others can be purchased for a nominal fee. To access this archive, go to **http://www.reutershealth.com/frame2/arch.html** and search by "thyroid cancer" (or synonyms). The following was recently listed in this archive for thyroid cancer:

- **Marine organism-derived aplidine advances against rare thyroid cancer**
  Source: Reuters Medical News
  Date: October 22, 2002
  http://www.reuters.gov/archive/2002/10/22/professional/links/20021022drgd002.html

- **Zeltia's aplidine advances against rare thyroid cancer**
  Source: Reuters Industry Breifing
  Date: October 21, 2002
  http://www.reuters.gov/archive/2002/10/21/business/links/20021021drgd006.html

- **Mortality low but recurrence high with thyroid cancer in children**
  Source: Reuters Medical News
  Date: August 29, 2002
  http://www.reuters.gov/archive/2002/08/29/professional/links/20020829clin005.html

- **UK guidelines aim to reduce thyroid cancer mortality**
  Source: Reuters Medical News
  Date: March 22, 2002
  http://www.reuters.gov/archive/2002/03/22/professional/links/20020322plcy002.html

- **UK guidelines aim to cut thyroid cancer mortality**
  Source: Reuters Health eLine
  Date: March 22, 2002
  http://www.reuters.gov/archive/2002/03/22/eline/links/20020322elin020.html

- **Thyroid cancer can present in youngsters who carry RET oncogene mutation**
  Source: Reuters Medical News
  Date: February 01, 2002
  http://www.reuters.gov/archive/2002/02/01/professional/links/20020201epid007.html

- **Reproductive, hormonal factors influence risk of thyroid cancer**
  Source: Reuters Medical News
  Date: January 21, 2002
  http://www.reuters.gov/archive/2002/01/21/professional/links/20020121epid001.html

- **Chernobyl's young have high rate of thyroid cancer**
  Source: Reuters Health eLine
  Date: December 10, 2001
  http://www.reuters.gov/archive/2001/12/10/eline/links/20011210elin007.html

- **Many thyroid cancer cases linked to Chernobyl**
  Source: Reuters Health eLine
  Date: October 23, 2001
  http://www.reuters.gov/archive/2001/10/23/eline/links/20011023elin027.html

- **Radiation therapy for breast cancer does not increase risk of thyroid cancer**
  Source: Reuters Industry Breifing
  Date: September 27, 2001
  http://www.reuters.gov/archive/2001/09/27/business/links/20010927clin015.html

- **Breast tumor radiation not tied to thyroid cancer**
  Source: Reuters Health eLine
  Date: September 25, 2001
  http://www.reuters.gov/archive/2001/09/25/eline/links/20010925elin004.html

- **Thyroid cancer therapy may up breast cancer risk**
  Source: Reuters Health eLine
  Date: July 26, 2001
  http://www.reuters.gov/archive/2001/07/26/eline/links/20010726elin012.html

- **Thyroid cancer is the major continuing health effect of Chernobyl disaster**
  Source: Reuters Medical News
  Date: April 27, 2001
  http://www.reuters.gov/archive/2001/04/27/professional/links/20010427epid012.html

- **New test improves the detection of recurrent thyroid cancer**
  Source: Reuters Medical News
  Date: November 13, 2000
  http://www.reuters.gov/archive/2000/11/13/professional/links/20001113clin005.html

- **Thyroid cancer patients treated with radioactive iodine not a threat to family**
  Source: Reuters Medical News
  Date: May 05, 2000
  http://www.reuters.gov/archive/2000/05/05/professional/links/20000505clin012.html

- **Family safe from thyroid cancer patient's radiation**
  Source: Reuters Health eLine
  Date: May 03, 2000
  http://www.reuters.gov/archive/2000/05/03/eline/links/20000503elin006.html

- **Embolization effective for vertebral metastases of thyroid cancer**
  Source: Reuters Medical News
  Date: March 27, 2000
  http://www.reuters.gov/archive/2000/03/27/professional/links/20000327clin006.html

- **Children at risk for thyroid cancer following radiation therapy**
  Source: Reuters Medical News
  Date: December 20, 1999
  http://www.reuters.gov/archive/1999/12/20/professional/links/19991220clin013.html

- **Recombinant human TSH alternative to thyroid hormone withdrawal for thyroid cancer follow-up**
  Source: Reuters Medical News
  Date: November 22, 1999
  http://www.reuters.gov/archive/1999/11/22/professional/links/19991122clin012.html

- **After Chernobyl, pediatric thyroid cancer incidence escalated in Ukraine**
  Source: Reuters Medical News
  Date: July 01, 1999
  http://www.reuters.gov/archive/1999/07/01/professional/links/19990701epid001.html

- **Child thyroid cancer rises 10-fold after Chernobyl**
  Source: Reuters Health eLine
  Date: June 30, 1999
  http://www.reuters.gov/archive/1999/06/30/eline/links/19990630elin010.html

- **Lithium improves I-131 uptake, retention in thyroid cancer patients**
  Source: Reuters Medical News
  Date: March 31, 1999
  http://www.reuters.gov/archive/1999/03/31/professional/links/19990331clin008.html

- **Scans help detect thyroid cancer recurrence**
  Source: Reuters Health eLine
  Date: February 19, 1999
  http://www.reuters.gov/archive/1999/02/19/eline/links/19990219elin006.html

- **Screening for thyroid cancer due to nuclear bomb tests not advisable**
  Source: Reuters Medical News
  Date: September 02, 1998
  http://www.reuters.gov/archive/1998/09/02/professional/links/19980902plcy001.html

- **Experts advise against thyroid cancer screening**
  Source: Reuters Health eLine
  Date: September 02, 1998
  http://www.reuters.gov/archive/1998/09/02/eline/links/19980902elin007.html

- **Conventional Method Still Best In Radioiodine Scanning For Thyroid Cancer**
  Source: Reuters Medical News
  Date: September 29, 1997
  http://www.reuters.gov/archive/1997/09/29/professional/links/19970929clin008.html
- **Increase In Thyroid Cancer In Children Of Chernobyl**
  Source: Reuters Medical News
  Date: November 22, 1995
  http://www.reuters.gov/archive/1995/11/22/professional/links/19951122epid001.html
- **Incidence Of Thyroid Cancer Quintupled In Chernobyl Area**
  Source: Reuters Medical News
  Date: June 01, 1995
  http://www.reuters.gov/archive/1995/06/01/professional/links/19950601epid002.html

The NIH

Within MEDLINEplus, the NIH has made an agreement with the New York Times Syndicate, the AP News Service, and Reuters to deliver news that can be browsed by the public. Search news releases at **http://www.nlm.nih.gov/medlineplus/alphanews_a.html.** MEDLINEplus allows you to browse across an alphabetical index. Or you can search by date at **http://www.nlm.nih.gov/medlineplus/newsbydate.html**. Often, news items are indexed by MEDLINEplus within their search engine.

Business Wire

Business Wire is similar to PR Newswire. To access this archive, simply go to **http://www.businesswire.com**. You can scan the news by industry category or company name.

Internet Wire

Internet Wire is more focused on technology than the other wires. To access this site, go to **http://www.internetwire.com** and use the "Search Archive" option. Type in "thyroid cancer" (or synonyms). As this service is oriented to technology, you may wish to search for press releases covering diagnostic procedures or tests that you may have read about.

Search Engines

Free-to-view news can also be found in the news section of your favorite search engines (see the health news page at Yahoo: **http://dir.yahoo.com/Health/News_and_Media/,** or use this Web site's general news search page **http://news.yahoo.com/.** Type in "thyroid cancer" (or synonyms). If you know the name of a company that is relevant to thyroid cancer, you can go to any stock trading Web site (such as **www.etrade.com**) and search for the company name there. News items across various news sources are reported on indicated hyperlinks.

BBC

Covering news from a more European perspective, the British Broadcasting Corporation (BBC) allows the public free access to their news archive located at **http://www.bbc.co.uk/**. Search by "thyroid cancer" (or synonyms).

Newsletters on Thyroid Cancer

Given their focus on current and relevant developments, newsletters are often more useful to patients than academic articles. You can find newsletters using the Combined Health Information Database (CHID). You will need to use the "Detailed Search" option. To access CHID, go directly to the following hyperlink: **http://chid.nih.gov/detail/detail.html**. Your investigation must limit the search to "Newsletter" and "thyroid cancer." Go to the bottom of the search page where "You may refine your search by." Select the dates and language that you prefer. For the format option, select "Newsletter." By making these selections and typing in "thyroid cancer" or synonyms into the "For these words:" box, you will only receive results on newsletters. The following list was generated using the options described above:

- **Cutaneous Lymphoma Network**

    Source: Cincinnati, OH: Cutaneous Lymphoma Network. 1994. 8 p. (average).

Contact: Available from Cutaneous Lymphoma Network. Department of Dermatology, University of Cincinnati, Attn: Judi Van Horn, 234 Goodman Street, Pav. A-3, Cincinnati, OH 45269-0523. (513) 558- 6955. Price: Free.

Summary: This newsletter is a forum to share insights about cutaneous lymphoma. Articles discuss treatment, medical issues, and coping with the disease.

Newsletter Articles

If you choose not to subscribe to a newsletter, you can nevertheless find references to newsletter articles. We recommend that you use the Combined Health Information Database, while limiting your search criteria to "newsletter articles." Again, you will need to use the "Detailed Search" option. Go directly to the following hyperlink: **http://chid.nih.gov/detail/detail.html**. Go to the bottom of the search page where "You may refine your search by." Select the dates and language that you prefer. For the format option, select "Newsletter Article."

By making these selections, and typing in "thyroid cancer" (or synonyms) into the "For these words:" box, you will only receive results on newsletter articles. You should check back periodically with this database as it is updated every 3 months.

Academic Periodicals Covering Thyroid Cancer

Academic periodicals can be a highly technical yet valuable source of information on thyroid cancer. We have compiled the following list of periodicals known to publish articles relating to thyroid cancer and which are currently indexed within the National Library of Medicine's PubMed database (follow hyperlinks to view more information, summaries, etc., for each). In addition to these sources, to keep current on articles written on thyroid cancer published by any of the periodicals listed below, you can simply follow the hyperlink indicated or go to the following Web site: **www.ncbi.nlm.nih.gov/pubmed**. Type the periodical's name into the search box to find the latest studies published.

If you want complete details about the historical contents of a periodical, you can also visit **http://www.ncbi.nlm.nih.gov/entrez/jrbrowser.cgi**. Here, type in the name of the journal or its abbreviation, and you will receive an index of published articles. At **http://locatorplus.gov/** you can retrieve more indexing information on medical periodicals (e.g. the name of the publisher). Select the button "Search LOCATORplus." Then type in the name of the journal and select the advanced search option "Journal Title Search." The following is a sample of periodicals which publish articles on thyroid cancer:

- **Acta Oto-Laryngologica. (Acta Otolaryngol)**
  http://www.ncbi.nlm.nih.gov/entrez/jrbrowser.cgi?field=0&regexp=Acta+Oto-Laryngologica&dispmax=20&dispstart=0

- **Bmj (Clinical Research Ed. . (BMJ)**
  http://www.ncbi.nlm.nih.gov/entrez/jrbrowser.cgi?field=0&regexp=Bmj+(Clinical+Research+Ed.+&dispmax=20&dispstart=0

- **British Journal of Cancer. (Br J Cancer)**
  http://www.ncbi.nlm.nih.gov/entrez/jrbrowser.cgi?field=0&regexp=British+Journal+of+Cancer&dispmax=20&dispstart=0

- **Clinical Chemistry. (Clin Chem)**
  http://www.ncbi.nlm.nih.gov/entrez/jrbrowser.cgi?field=0&regexp=Clinical+Chemistry&dispmax=20&dispstart=0

- **Clinical Endocrinology. (Clin Endocrinol (Oxf))**
  http://www.ncbi.nlm.nih.gov/entrez/jrbrowser.cgi?field=0&regexp=Clinical+Endocrinology&dispmax=20&dispstart=0

- **Clinical Nuclear Medicine. (Clin Nucl Med)**
  http://www.ncbi.nlm.nih.gov/entrez/jrbrowser.cgi?field=0&regexp=Clinical+Nuclear+Medicine&dispmax=20&dispstart=0

- **Experimental and Clinical Endocrinology & Diabetes : Official Journal, German Society of Endocrinology [and] German Diabetes Association. (Exp Clin Endocrinol Diabetes)**
  http://www.ncbi.nlm.nih.gov/entrez/jrbrowser.cgi?field=0&regexp=Experimental+and+Clinical+Endocrinology+&+Diabetes+:+Official+Journal,+German+Society+of+Endocrinology+[and]+German+Diabetes+Association&dispmax=20&dispstart=0

- **Journal of Surgical Oncology. (J Surg Oncol)**
  http://www.ncbi.nlm.nih.gov/entrez/jrbrowser.cgi?field=0&regexp=Journal+of+Surgical+Oncology&dispmax=20&dispstart=0

- **Molecular Endocrinology (Baltimore, Md. . (Mol Endocrinol)**
  http://www.ncbi.nlm.nih.gov/entrez/jrbrowser.cgi?field=0&regexp=Molecular+Endocrinology+(Baltimore,+Md.+&dispmax=20&dispstart=0

- **Surgical Oncology. (Surg Oncol)**
  http://www.ncbi.nlm.nih.gov/entrez/jrbrowser.cgi?field=0&regexp=Surgical+Oncology&dispmax=20&dispstart=0

- **The Journal of Laryngology and Otology. (J Laryngol Otol)**
  http://www.ncbi.nlm.nih.gov/entrez/jrbrowser.cgi?field=0&regexp=The+Journal+of+Laryngology+and+Otology&dispmax=20&dispstart=0

- **The Journal of Otolaryngology. (J Otolaryngol)**
  http://www.ncbi.nlm.nih.gov/entrez/jrbrowser.cgi?field=0&regexp=The+Journal+of+Otolaryngology&dispmax=20&dispstart=0

Vocabulary Builder

Amyloidosis: A group of diseases in which protein is deposited in specific organs (localized amyloidosis) or throughout the body (systemic amyloidosis). Amyloidosis may be either primary (with no known cause) or secondary (caused by another disease, including some types of cancer). Generally, primary amyloidosis affects the nerves, skin, tongue, joints, heart, and liver; secondary amyloidosis often affects the spleen, kidneys, liver, and adrenal glands. [NIH]

Androgenic: Producing masculine characteristics. [EU]

Angiogenesis: Blood vessel formation. Tumor angiogenesis is the growth of blood vessels from surrounding tissue to a solid tumor. This is caused by the release of chemicals by the tumor. [NIH]

Aplidine: An anticancer drug obtained from a marine animal. [NIH]

Aqueous: Having to do with water. [NIH]

Chronic: A disease or condition that persists or progresses over a long period of time. [NIH]

Collagen: A fibrous protein found in cartilage and other connective tissue.

[NIH]

Dermatology: A medical specialty concerned with the skin, its structure, functions, diseases, and treatment. [NIH]

Docetaxel: An anticancer drug that belongs to the family of drugs called mitotic inhibitors. [NIH]

Dysplasia: Cells that look abnormal under a microscope but are not cancer. [NIH]

Elasticity: Resistance and recovery from distortion of shape. [NIH]

Flavopiridol: Belongs to the family of anticancer drugs called flavinols. [NIH]

Gallium: A rare, metallic element designated by the symbol, Ga, atomic number 31, and atomic weight 69.72. [NIH]

Gastrointestinal: Refers to the stomach and intestines. [NIH]

Gliadin: Simple protein, one of the prolamines, derived from the gluten of wheat, rye, etc. May be separated into 4 discrete electrophoretic fractions. It is the toxic factor associated with celiac disease. [NIH]

Glutamine: An amino acid used in nutrition therapy. It is also being studied for the treatment of diarrhea caused by radiation therapy to the pelvis. [NIH]

Gluten: The protein of wheat and other grains which gives to the dough its tough elastic character. [EU]

Grasses: A large family, gramineae, of narrow-leaved herbaceous monocots. Many grasses produce highly allergenic pollens and are hosts to cattle parasites and toxic fungi. [NIH]

Hematology: A subspecialty of internal medicine concerned with morphology, physiology, and pathology of the blood and blood-forming tissues. [NIH]

Immunotherapy: Treatment to stimulate or restore the ability of the immune system to fight infection and disease. Also used to lessen side effects that may be caused by some cancer treatments. Also called biological therapy or biological response modifier (BRM) therapy. [NIH]

Irinotecan: An anticancer drug that belongs to a family of anticancer drugs called topoisomerase inhibitors. It is a camptothecin analogue. Also called CPT 11. [NIH]

Lubricants: Oily or slippery substances. [NIH]

Lymphocyte: A white blood cell. Lymphocytes have a number of roles in the immune system, including the production of antibodies and other substances that fight infection and diseases. [NIH]

Lymphoid: Referring to lymphocytes, a type of white blood cell. Also refers to tissue in which lymphocytes develop. [NIH]

Molecule: A chemical made up of two or more atoms. The atoms in a molecule can be the same (an oxygen molecule has two oxygen atoms) or different (a water molecule has two hydrogen atoms and one oxygen atom). Biological molecules, such as proteins and DNA, can be made up of many thousands of atoms. [NIH]

Nausea: An unpleasant sensation, vaguely referred to the epigastrium and abdomen, and often culminating in vomiting. [EU]

Neurologic: Having to do with nerves or the nervous system. [NIH]

Ointments: Semisolid preparations used topically for protective emollient effects or as a vehicle for local administration of medications. Ointment bases are various mixtures of fats, waxes, animal and plant oils and solid and liquid hydrocarbons. [NIH]

Preclinical: Before a disease becomes clinically recognizable. [EU]

Proline: A non-essential amino acid that is synthesized from glutamic acid. It is an essential component of collagen and is important for proper functioning of joints and tendons. [NIH]

Sarcoidosis: An idiopathic systemic inflammatory granulomatous disorder comprised of epithelioid and multinucleated giant cells with little necrosis. It usually invades the lungs with fibrosis and may also involve lymph nodes, skin, liver, spleen, eyes, phalangeal bones, and parotid glands. [NIH]

Vascular: Pertaining to blood vessels or indicative of a copious blood supply. [EU]

Vertebral: Of or pertaining to a vertebra. [EU]

CHAPTER 8. PHYSICIAN GUIDELINES AND DATABASES

Overview

Doctors and medical researchers rely on a number of information sources to help patients with their conditions. Many will subscribe to journals or newsletters published by their professional associations or refer to specialized textbooks or clinical guides published for the medical profession. In this chapter, we focus on databases and Internet-based guidelines created or written for this professional audience.

NIH Guidelines

For the more common diseases, The National Institutes of Health publish guidelines that are frequently consulted by physicians. Publications are typically written by one or more of the various NIH Institutes. For physician guidelines, commonly referred to as "clinical" or "professional" guidelines, you can visit the following Institutes:

- Office of the Director (OD); guidelines consolidated across agencies available at **http://www.nih.gov/health/consumer/conkey.htm**

- National Institute of General Medical Sciences (NIGMS); fact sheets available at **http://www.nigms.nih.gov/news/facts/**

- National Library of Medicine (NLM); extensive encyclopedia (A.D.A.M., Inc.) with guidelines:
  http://www.nlm.nih.gov/medlineplus/healthtopics.html

- National Cancer Institute (NCI); guidelines available at
  http://cancernet.nci.nih.gov/pdq/pdq_treatment.shtml

In this chapter, we begin by reproducing one such guideline for thyroid cancer:

What Is Thyroid Cancer?[32]

Carcinoma of the thyroid gland is an uncommon cancer but, nonetheless, is the most common malignancy of the endocrine system.[33] Differentiated tumors (papillary or follicular) are highly treatable and usually curable. Poorly differentiated cancers (medullary or anaplastic) are much less common, are aggressive, metastasize early, and have a much poorer prognosis. Thyroid cancer affects women more commonly than men, and the majority of cases occur in patients between the ages of 25 and 65. The incidence of this malignancy has been increasing over the last decade. The prognosis for differentiated carcinoma is better for patients younger than 40 years of age without extracapsular extension or vascular invasion.[34] Age appears to be the single most important prognostic factor.[35] Thyroid cancer commonly presents as a cold nodule. The overall incidence of cancer in a cold nodule is 12% to 15%, but it is higher in patients under 40 years of age.[36]

The prognostic significance of lymph node status is controversial. One retrospective surgical series of 931 previously untreated patients with differentiated thyroid cancer found that female gender, multifocality, and regional node involvement are favorable prognostic factors.[37] Adverse

---

[32] The following guidelines appeared on the NCI website on Aug 26, 2002. The text was last modified Jul, 2002. The text has been adapted for this sourcebook.

[33] Hundahl SA, Fleming ID, Fremgen AM, et al.: A National Cancer Data Base report on 53,856 cases of thyroid carcinoma treated in the U.S., 1985-1995. Cancer 83(12): 2638-2648, 1998.

[34] Grant CS, Hay ID, Gough IR, et al.: Local recurrence in papillary thyroid carcinoma: Is extent of surgical resection important? Surgery 104(6): 954-962, 1988.
Sanders LE, Cady B: Differentiated thyroid cancer: reexamination of risk groups and outcome of treatment. Archives of Surgery 133(4): 419-425, 1998.
Mazzaferri EL: Treating differentiated thyroid carcinoma: where do we draw the line? Mayo Clinic Proceedings 66(1): 105-111, 1991.
Staunton MD: Thyroid cancer: a multivariate analysis on influence of treatment on long-term survival. European Journal of Surgical Oncology 20: 613-621, 1994.
Mazzaferri EL, Jhiang SM: Long-term impact of initial surgical and medical therapy on papillary and follicular thyroid cancer. American Journal of Medicine 97: 418-428, 1994.

[35] Mazzaferri EL: Treating differentiated thyroid carcinoma: where do we draw the line? Mayo Clinic Proceedings 66(1): 105-111, 1991.

[36] Tennvall J, Biorklund A, Moller T, et al.: Is the EORTC prognostic index of thyroid cancer valid in differentiated thyroid carcinoma?: retrospective multivariate analysis of differentiated thyroid carcinoma with long follow-up. Cancer 57(7): 1405-1414, 1986.

[37] Shah JP, Loree TR, Dharker D, et al.: Prognostic factors in differentiated carcinoma of the thyroid gland. American Journal of Surgery 164(6): 658-661, 1992.

factors included age over 45 years, follicular histology, primary greater than 4 centimeters (T2-3), extrathyroid extension (T4), and distant metastases.[38] Other studies, however, have shown that regional lymph node involvement had no effect[39] or even an adverse effect on survival.[40] Diffuse, intense immunostaining for vascular endothelial growth factor in patients with papillary cancer has been associated with a high rate of local recurrence and distant metastases.[41] An elevated serum thyroglobulin level correlates strongly with recurrent tumor when found in patients with differentiated thyroid cancer during postoperative evaluations.[42] Serum thyroglobulin levels are most sensitive when patients are hypothyroid and have elevated serum thyroid-stimulating hormone levels.[43] Expression of the tumor suppressor gene p53 has also been associated with an adverse prognosis for patients with thyroid cancer.[44]

Patients considered to be low-risk by the age, metastases, extent, and size (AMES) risk criteria include women younger than 50 years of age and men younger than 40 years of age without evidence of distant metastases. Also included in the low-risk group are older patients with primary tumors less

---

[38] Shah JP, Loree TR, Dharker D, et al.: Prognostic factors in differentiated carcinoma of the thyroid gland. American Journal of Surgery 164(6): 658-661, 1992.
Andersen PE, Kinsella J, Loree TR, et al.: Differentiated carcinoma of the thyroid with extrathyroidal extension. American Journal of Surgery 170(5): 467-470, 1995.
[39] Coburn MC, Wanebo HJ: Prognostic factors and management considerations in patients with cervical metastases of thyroid cancer. American Journal of Surgery 164(6): 671-676, 1992.
[40] Staunton MD: Thyroid cancer: a multivariate analysis on influence of treatment on long-term survival. European Journal of Surgical Oncology 20: 613-621, 1994.
Mazzaferri EL, Jhiang SM: Long-term impact of initial surgical and medical therapy on papillary and follicular thyroid cancer. American Journal of Medicine 97: 418-428, 1994.
Sellers M, Beenken S, Blankenship A, et al.: Prognostic significance of cervical lymph node metastases in differentiated thyroid cancer. American Journal of Surgery 164(6): 578-581, 1992.
[41] Lennard CM, Patel A, Wilson J, et al.: Intensity of vascular endothelial growth factor expression is associated with increased risk of recurrence and decreased disease-free survival in papillary thyroid cancer. Surgery 129(5): 552-558, 2001.
[42] van Herle AJ, van Herle KA: Thyroglobulin in benign and malignant thyroid disease. In: Falk SA: Thyroid disease: endocrinology, surgery, nuclear medicine, and radiotherapy. Philadelphia: Lippincott-Raven, 1997, pp 601-618.
Ruiz-Garcia J, Ruiz de Almodovar JM, Olea N, et al.: Thyroglobulin level as a predictive factor of tumoral recurrence in differentiated thyroid cancer. Journal of Nuclear Medicine 32(3): 395-398, 1991.
[43] Duren M, Siperstein AE, Shen W, et al.: Value of stimulated serum thyroglobulin levels for detecting persistent or recurrent differentiated thyroid cancer in high- and low-risk patients. Surgery 126(1): 13-19, 1999.
[44] Godballe C, Asschenfeldt P, Jorgensen KE, et al.: Prognostic factors in papillary and follicular thyroid carcinomas: p53 expression is a significant indicator of prognosis. Laryngoscope 108(2): 243-249, 1998.

than 5 centimeters and papillary cancer without evidence of gross extrathyroid invasion or follicular cancer without either major capsular invasion or blood vessel invasion.[45] Using these criteria, a retrospective study of 1019 patients showed that the 20-year survival rate is 98% for low-risk patients and 50% for high-risk patients.[46]

Patients with a history of radiation administered in infancy and childhood for benign conditions of the head and neck, such as enlarged thymus, acne, or tonsillar or adenoidal enlargement have an increased risk of cancer as well as other abnormalities of the thyroid gland. In this group of patients, malignancies of the thyroid gland first appear beginning as early as 5 years following radiation and may appear 20 or more years later.[47] Other risk factors for the development of thyroid cancer include a history of goiter, family history of thyroid disease, female gender, and Asian race.[48] The thyroid gland may occasionally be the site of other primary tumors, including sarcomas, lymphomas, epidermoid carcinomas, and teratoma, and may be the site of metastasis from other cancers, particularly of the lung, breast, and kidney.

Cellular Classification

Cell type is an important determinant of prognosis in thyroid cancer. There are 4 main varieties of thyroid cancer (although, for clinical management of the patient, thyroid cancer is generally divided into well-differentiated or poorly differentiated):[49]

    a) papillary carcinoma
        papillary/follicular carcinoma
    b) follicular carcinoma
        Hurthle cell carcinoma
    c) medullary carcinoma

---

[45] Sanders LE, Cady B: Differentiated thyroid cancer: reexamination of risk groups and outcome of treatment. Archives of Surgery 133(4): 419-425, 1998.
[46] Sanders LE, Cady B: Differentiated thyroid cancer: reexamination of risk groups and outcome of treatment. Archives of Surgery 133(4): 419-425, 1998.
[47] Fraker DL, Skarulis M, Livolsi V: Thyroid tumors. In: DeVita VT Jr, Hellman S, Rosenberg SA, eds.: Cancer: Principles and Practice of Oncology. Philadelphia, Pa: Lippincott-Raven Publishers, 5th ed., 1997, pp 1629-1652.
[48] Iribarren C, Haselkorn T, Tekawa IS, et al.: Cohort study of thyroid cancer in San Francisco bay area population. International Journal of Cancer 93(5): 745-750, 2001.
[49] LiVolsi VA: Pathology of thyroid disease. In: Falk SA: Thyroid disease: endocrinology, surgery, nuclear medicine, and radiotherapy. Philadelphia: Lippincott-Raven, 1997, pp 127-175.

d) anaplastic carcinoma
   small cell carcinoma
   giant cell carcinoma
e) others
   lymphoma
   sarcoma
   carcinosarcoma

A definition for each major type can be found under stage information.

Stage Information

The American Joint Committee on Cancer (AJCC) has designated staging by TNM classification.[50]

TNM Definitions

Primary Tumor (T)[51]

- TX: Primary tumor cannot be assessed
- T0: No evidence of primary tumor
- T1: Tumor 1 cm or less in greatest dimension limited to the thyroid
- T2: Tumor more than 1 cm but not more than 4 cm in greatest dimension limited to the thyroid
- T3: Tumor more than 4 cm in greatest dimension limited to the thyroid
- T4: Tumor of any size extending beyond the thyroid capsule

Regional Lymph Nodes (N)

Regional lymph nodes are the cervical and upper mediastinal lymph nodes.

- NX: Regional lymph nodes cannot be assessed
- N0: No regional lymph node metastasis

---

[50] Thyroid Gland. In: American Joint Committee on Cancer: AJCC Cancer Staging Manual. Philadelphia, Pa: Lippincott-Raven Publishers, 5th ed., 1997, pp 59-64.
[51] Note: All categories may be subdivided into (a) solitary tumor or (b) multifocal tumor (the largest determines the classification).

- N1: Regional lymph node metastasis
  - N1a: Metastasis in ipsilateral cervical lymph node(s)
  - N1b: Metastasis in bilateral, midline, or contralateral cervical or mediastinal lymph node(s)

Distant Metastases (M)

- MX: Distant metastasis cannot be assessed
- M0: No distant metastasis
- M1: Distant metastasis

AJCC Stage Groupings for Papillary or Follicular

Under 45 Years

Stage I:
- Any T, Any N, M0

Stage II:
- Any T, Any N, M1

45 Years and Older

Stage I:
- T1, N0, M0

Stage II:
- T2, N0, M0
- T3, N0, M0

Stage III:
- T4, N0, M0
- Any T, N1, M0

Stage IV:

- Any T, Any N, M1

AJCC Stage Groupings for Medullary

Stage I:

- T1, N0, M0

Stage II:

- T2, N0, M0
- T3, N0, M0
- T4, N0, M0

Stage III:

- Any T, N1, M0

Stage IV:

- Any T, Any N, M1

AJCC Stage Groupings for Undifferentiated (Anaplastic)

All cases are stage IV.

Stage IV:

- Any T, Any N, Any M

Papillary Staging

Stage I Papillary

Stage I papillary carcinoma is localized to the thyroid gland. In as many as 50% of cases there are multifocal sites of papillary adenocarcinomas throughout the gland. Most papillary cancers have some follicular elements, and these may sometimes be more numerous than the papillary formations, but this does not change the prognosis. The 10-year survival rate is slightly better for patients younger than 40 years of age than for patients older than 40 years of age.

Stage II Papillary

Stage II papillary carcinoma is defined as either 1) tumor that has spread distantly in patients younger than 45 years of age or 2) tumor that is greater than 1 centimeter in size and is limited to the thyroid gland in patients older than 45 years of age. In as many as 50% to 80% of cases there are multifocal sites of papillary adenocarcinomas throughout the gland. Most papillary cancers have some follicular elements, and these may sometimes be more numerous than the papillary formations, but this does not appear to change the prognosis.

Stage III Papillary

Stage III is papillary carcinoma in patients older than 45 years of age with local cervical invasion or positive lymph nodes. Papillary carcinoma which has invaded adjacent cervical tissue has a worse prognosis than tumors confined to the thyroid.

Stage IV Papillary

Stage IV is papillary carcinoma in patients older than 45 years of age with distant metastases. The lungs and bone are the most frequent distant sites of spread, although such distant spread is rare in this type of thyroid cancer. Papillary carcinoma more frequently metastasizes to regional lymph nodes than to distant sites. The prognosis for patients with distant metastases is poor.

Follicular Staging

Stage I Follicular

Stage I follicular carcinoma is localized to the thyroid gland. Follicular thyroid carcinoma must be distinguished from follicular adenomas, which are characterized by their lack of invasion through the capsule into the surrounding thyroid tissue. While follicular cancers have a good prognosis, it is less favorable than that of papillary carcinoma. The 10-year survival for patients with follicular carcinoma without vascular invasion is better than for patients with vascular invasion.

Stage II Follicular

Stage II follicular carcinoma is defined as either; tumor that has spread distantly in patients younger than 45 years of age, or tumor that is greater than 1 centimeter in size and is limited to the thyroid gland in patients older than 45 years of age. The presence of lymph node metastases does not worsen the prognosis. Follicular thyroid carcinoma must be distinguished from follicular adenomas, which are characterized by their lack of invasion through the capsule into the surrounding thyroid tissue. While follicular cancers have a good prognosis, it is less favorable than that of papillary carcinoma; the 10-year survival for patients with follicular carcinoma without vascular invasion is better than for patients with vascular invasion.

Stage III Follicular

Stage III is follicular carcinoma in patients older than 45 years of age with local cervical invasion or positive lymph nodes. Follicular carcinoma invading cervical tissue has a worse prognosis than tumors confined to the thyroid gland. The presence of vascular invasion is an additional poor prognostic factor. Metastases to lymph nodes do not worsen the prognosis.

Stage IV Follicular

Stage IV is follicular carcinoma in patients older than 45 years of age with distant metastases. The lungs and bone are the most frequent sites of spread. Follicular carcinomas more commonly have blood vessel invasion and tend to metastasize hematogenously to the lungs and to the bone rather than through the lymphatic system. The prognosis for patients with distant metastases is poor.

Medullary Staging

Several staging systems have been employed to correlate extent of disease with long-term survival in medullary thyroid cancer. The clinical staging system of the AJCC correlates survival to size of the primary tumor, presence or absence of lymph node metastases, and presence or absence of distance metastasis. Patients with the best prognosis are those who are diagnosed by provocative screening, prior to the appearance of palpable disease.[52]

Stage I Medullary

Tumor less than 1 cm in size or clinically occult disease detected by provocative biochemical screening.

Stage II Medullary

Tumor greater than 1 cm but less than 4 cm.

Stage III Medullary

Lymph node metastasis.

Stage IV medullary

Distant metastasis (any T, any N, M1).

Medullary carcinoma usually presents as a hard mass, and is often accompanied by blood vessel invasion. Medullary thyroid cancer occurs in 2 forms: sporadic and familial. In the sporadic form the tumor is usually unilateral. In the familial form, the tumor is almost always bilateral. In addition, the familial form may be associated with benign or malignant tumors of other endocrine organs, commonly referred to as the multiple endocrine neoplasia syndromes (MEN 2A or MEN 2B).

In this syndrome, there is an association with pheochromocytoma of the adrenal gland and parathyroid hyperplasia. Medullary carcinoma usually secretes calcitonin, a hormonal marker for the tumor, and may be detectable in blood even though the tumor is clinically occult. Metastases to regional lymph nodes are found in about 50% of cases. Prognosis depends on extent

---

[52] Colson YL, Carty SE: Medullary thyroid carcinoma. American Journal of Otolaryngology 14(2): 73-81, 1993.

of disease at presentation, presence or absence of regional lymph node metastases, and completeness of the surgical resection.[53]

Family members should be screened for calcitonin elevation to identify individuals who are at risk of developing familial medullary thyroid cancer. MEN 2A gene carrier status can be more accurately determined by analysis of mutations in the RET gene. Whereas modest elevation of calcitonin may lead to a false-positive diagnosis of medullary carcinoma, DNA testing for the RET mutation is the optimal approach in evaluating MEN 2A. All patients with medullary carcinoma of the thyroid (whether familial or sporadic) should be tested for RET mutations, and if they are positive, then family members should also be tested. Family members who are gene carriers should undergo prophylactic thyroidectomy at an early age.[54]

Anaplastic Staging

There is no generally accepted staging system for anaplastic thyroid cancer. All patients are considered to have stage IV disease.

Undifferentiated (anaplastic) carcinoma tumors are highly malignant cancers of the thyroid. They may be subclassified as small cell or large cell carcinomas. Both grow rapidly and extend to structures beyond the thyroid. Both small cell and large cell carcinoma present as hard, ill-defined masses, often with extension into the structures surrounding the thyroid. Small cell anaplastic thyroid carcinoma must be carefully distinguished from lymphoma. This tumor usually occurs in an older age group and is characterized by extensive local invasion and rapid progression. Five-year survival with this tumor is poor. Death is usually from uncontrolled local cancer in the neck, usually within months of diagnosis.

---

[53] Fraker DL, Skarulis M, Livolsi V: Thyroid tumors. In: DeVita VT Jr, Hellman S, Rosenberg SA, eds.: Cancer: Principles and Practice of Oncology. Philadelphia, Pa: Lippincott-Raven Publishers, 5th ed., 1997, pp 1629-1652.
[54] Lips CJ, Landsvater RM, Hoppener JW, et al.: Clinical screening as compared with DNA analysis in families with multiple endocrine neoplasia type 2A. New England Journal of Medicine 331(13): 828-835, 1994.
Decker RA, Peacock ML, Borst MJ, et al.: Progress in genetic screening of multiple endocrine neoplasia type 2A: is calcitonin testing obsolete? Surgery 118(2): 257-264, 1995.

Treatment Option Overview

The designations in PDQ that treatments are "standard" or "under clinical evaluation" are not to be used as a basis for reimbursement determinations.

Stage I Papillary Thyroid Cancer

Surgery is the therapy of choice for all primary lesions. Surgical options include total thyroidectomy or lobectomy. The choice of procedure is influenced mainly by the age of the patient and the size of the nodule. Survival results may be similar; the difference between them lies in the rates of surgical complications and local recurrences.[55]

Standard Treatment Options

Lobectomy:

- This procedure is associated with a lower incidence of complications, but approximately 5% to 10% of patients will have a recurrence in the thyroid following lobectomy.[56] Patients younger than 45 years of age will have the longest follow-up period and the greatest opportunity for recurrence. Abnormal regional lymph nodes should be biopsied at the time of surgery. Recognized nodal involvement should be removed at initial surgery but selective node removal can be performed and radical neck dissection is not required.

- Following the surgical procedure, patients should receive postoperative treatment with exogenous thyroid hormone in doses sufficient to

---

[55] Fraker DL, Skarulis M, Livolsi V: Thyroid tumors. In: DeVita VT Jr, Hellman S, Rosenberg SA, eds.: Cancer: Principles and Practice of Oncology. Philadelphia, Pa: Lippincott-Raven Publishers, 5th ed., 1997, pp 1629-1652.
Grant CS, Hay ID, Gough IR, et al.: Local recurrence in papillary thyroid carcinoma: Is extent of surgical resection important? Surgery 104(6): 954-962, 1988.
Cady B, Rossi R: An expanded view of risk-group definition in differentiated thyroid carcinoma. Surgery 104(6): 947-953, 1988.
Mazzaferri EL, Jhiang SM: Long-term impact of initial surgical and medical therapy on papillary and follicular thyroid cancer. American Journal of Medicine 97: 418-428, 1994.
Staunton MD: Thyroid cancer: a multivariate analysis on influence of treatment on long-term survival. European Journal of Surgical Oncology 20: 613-621, 1994.
[56] Hay ID, Grant CS, Bergstralh EJ, et al.: Unilateral total lobectomy: is it sufficient surgical treatment for patients with AMES low-risk papillary thyroid carcinoma? Surgery 124(6): 958-964; discussion 964-966, 1998.

suppress thyroid-stimulating hormone, since studies have shown a decreased incidence of recurrence.

I-131:

- Studies have shown that a postoperative course of therapeutic (ablative) doses of I-131 results in a decreased recurrence rate in papillary and follicular carcinomas.[57] It may be given in addition to exogenous thyroid hormone, but is not considered routine.[58] Patients presenting with papillary thyroid microcarcinomas (tumors <10 mm) have an excellent prognosis when treated surgically, and additional therapy with I-131 would not be expected to improve the prognosis.[59]

Total thyroidectomy:

- This procedure is advocated because of the high incidence of multicentric involvement of both lobes of the gland and the question of de-differentiation of the residual tumor to the anaplastic cell type. The procedure is associated with a higher incidence of hypoparathyroidism, but this complication may be reduced when a small amount of tissue remains on the contralateral side. This approach facilitates follow-up thyroid scanning.

Stage I Follicular Thyroid Cancer

Surgery is the therapy of choice for all primary lesions. Surgical options include total thyroidectomy or lobectomy. The age of the patient and the size of the nodule influence the selection of the operative procedure. Survival results are similar; the difference between them lies in the rates of surgical complications and local recurrences.[60]

---

[57] Mazzaferri EL, Jhiang SM: Long-term impact of initial surgical and medical therapy on papillary and follicular thyroid cancer. American Journal of Medicine 97: 418-428, 1994.

[58] Beierwaltes WH, Rabbani R, Dmuchowski C, et al.: An analysis of "Ablation of Thyroid Remnants" with I-131 in 511 patients from 1947-1984: experience at University of Michigan. Journal of Nuclear Medicine 25(12): 1287-1293, 1984.

[59] Hay ID, Grant CS, van Heerden JA, et al.: Papillary thyroid microcarcinoma: a study of 535 cases observed in a 50-year period. Surgery 112(6): 1139-1147, 1992.

[60] Fraker DL, Skarulis M, Livolsi V: Thyroid tumors. In: DeVita VT Jr, Hellman S, Rosenberg SA, eds.: Cancer: Principles and Practice of Oncology. Philadelphia, Pa: Lippincott-Raven Publishers, 5th ed., 1997, pp 1629-1652.

Tollefsen HR, Shah JP, Huvos AG: Follicular carcinoma of the thyroid. American Journal of Surgery 126(4): 523-528, 1973.

Edis AJ: Surgical treatment for thyroid cancer. Surgical Clinics of North America 57(3): 533-542, 1977.

Standard Treatment Options

Total thyroidectomy:

- This procedure is advocated because of the high incidence of multicentric involvement of both lobes of the gland. However, it is associated with a higher incidence of hypoparathyroidism. This complication may be reduced when a small amount of tissue remains on the contralateral side. This approach facilitates follow-up thyroid scanning.

Lobectomy:

- This procedure is associated with a lower incidence of complications, but approximately 5% to 10% of patients will have a recurrence in the thyroid following lobectomy. Follicular thyroid cancer commonly metastasizes to lung and bone; with a remnant lobe in place, use of I-131 as ablative therapy is compromised. Abnormal regional lymph nodes should be biopsied at the time of surgery. Recognized nodal involvement should be removed at initial surgery but selective node removal can be performed and radical neck dissection is not required.

- Following the surgical procedure, patients should receive postoperative treatment with exogenous thyroid hormone in doses sufficient to suppress thyroid-stimulating hormone, since studies have shown a decreased incidence of recurrence.

I-131:

- Studies have shown that a postoperative course of therapeutic (ablative) doses of I-131 results in a decreased recurrence rate in papillary and follicular carcinomas.[61] It should be given in addition to exogenous thyroid hormone.[62]

Staunton MD: Thyroid cancer: a multivariate analysis on influence of treatment on long-term survival. European Journal of Surgical Oncology 20: 613-621, 1994.
Mazzaferri EL, Jhiang SM: Long-term impact of initial surgical and medical therapy on papillary and follicular thyroid cancer. American Journal of Medicine 97: 418-428, 1994.
[61] Mazzaferri EL, Jhiang SM: Long-term impact of initial surgical and medical therapy on papillary and follicular thyroid cancer. American Journal of Medicine 97: 418-428, 1994.
[62] Beierwaltes WH, Rabbani R, Dmuchowski C, et al.: An analysis of "Ablation of Thyroid Remnants" with I-131 in 511 patients from 1947-1984: experience at University of Michigan. Journal of Nuclear Medicine 25(12): 1287-1293, 1984.

Stage II Papillary Thyroid Cancer

Surgery is the therapy of choice for all primary lesions. Surgical options include total thyroidectomy or lobectomy. The choice of procedure is influenced mainly by the age of the patient and the size of the nodule. Survival results may be similar; the difference between them lies in the rates of surgical complications and local recurrences.[63]

Standard Treatment Options

Lobectomy:

- This procedure is associated with a lower incidence of complications, but approximately 5% to 10% of patients will have a recurrence in the thyroid following lobectomy. Patients under the age of 45 will have the longest follow-up period and the greatest opportunity for recurrence. Abnormal regional lymph nodes should be biopsied at the time of surgery. Recognized nodal involvement should be removed at initial surgery but selective node removal can be performed and radical neck dissection is not required. This results in a decreased recurrence rate, but has not been shown to improve survival.

- Following the surgical procedure, patients should receive postoperative treatment with exogenous thyroid hormone in doses sufficient to suppress thyroid-stimulating hormone, since studies have shown a decreased incidence of recurrence.

I-131:

- Studies have shown that a postoperative course of therapeutic (ablative) doses of I-131 results in a decreased recurrence rate in papillary and

---

[63] Fraker DL, Skarulis M, Livolsi V: Thyroid tumors. In: DeVita VT Jr, Hellman S, Rosenberg SA, eds.: Cancer: Principles and Practice of Oncology. Philadelphia, Pa: Lippincott-Raven Publishers, 5th ed., 1997, pp 1629-1652.
Grant CS, Hay ID, Gough IR, et al.: Local recurrence in papillary thyroid carcinoma: Is extent of surgical resection important? Surgery 104(6): 954-962, 1988.
Cady B, Rossi R: An expanded view of risk-group definition in differentiated thyroid carcinoma. Surgery 104(6): 947-953, 1988.
Staunton MD: Thyroid cancer: a multivariate analysis on influence of treatment on long-term survival. European Journal of Surgical Oncology 20: 613-621, 1994.
Mazzaferri EL, Jhiang SM: Long-term impact of initial surgical and medical therapy on papillary and follicular thyroid cancer. American Journal of Medicine 97: 418-428, 1994.

follicular carcinomas.[64] It may be given in addition to exogenous thyroid hormone, but is not considered routine.[65]

Total thyroidectomy:

- This procedure is advocated because of the high incidence of multicentric involvement of both lobes of the gland and the question of de-differentiation of the residual tumor to the anaplastic cell type. The procedure is associated with a higher incidence of hypoparathyroidism, but this complication may be reduced when a small amount of tissue remains on the contralateral side. This approach facilitates follow-up thyroid scanning.

Stage II Follicular Thyroid Cancer

Surgery is the therapy of choice for all primary lesions. Surgical options include near total thyroidectomy and lobectomy. The age of the patient and the size of the nodule influence the selection of the operative procedure. Survival results are similar; the difference between them lies in the rates of surgical complications and local recurrences.[66]

Standard Treatment Options

Total thyroidectomy:

- This procedure is advocated because of the high incidence of multicentric involvement of both lobes of the gland. However, it is associated with a higher incidence of hypoparathyroidism. This complication is reduced when a small amount of tissue remains on the contralateral side. This approach facilitates follow-up thyroid scanning.

---

[64] Mazzaferri EL, Jhiang SM: Long-term impact of initial surgical and medical therapy on papillary and follicular thyroid cancer. American Journal of Medicine 97: 418-428, 1994.
[65] Beierwaltes WH, Rabbani R, Dmuchowski C, et al.: An analysis of "Ablation of Thyroid Remnants" with I-131 in 511 patients from 1947-1984: experience at University of Michigan. Journal of Nuclear Medicine 25(12): 1287-1293, 1984.
[66] Fraker DL, Skarulis M, Livolsi V: Thyroid tumors. In: DeVita VT Jr, Hellman S, Rosenberg SA, eds.: Cancer: Principles and Practice of Oncology. Philadelphia, Pa: Lippincott-Raven Publishers, 5th ed., 1997, pp 1629-1652.
Tollefsen HR, Shah JP, Huvos AG: Follicular carcinoma of the thyroid. American Journal of Surgery 126(4): 523-528, 1973.
Edis AJ: Surgical treatment for thyroid cancer. Surgical Clinics of North America 57(3): 533-542, 1977.

Lobectomy:

- This procedure is associated with a lower incidence of complications, but approximately 5% to 10% of patients will have a recurrence in the thyroid following lobectomy. Follicular thyroid cancer commonly metastasizes to lung and bone; with a remnant lobe in place, use of I-131 as ablative therapy is compromised. Abnormal regional lymph nodes should be biopsied at the time of surgery. Recognized nodal involvement should be removed at initial surgery but selective node removal can be performed and radical node dissection is not required.

- Following the surgical procedure, patients should receive postoperative treatment with exogenous thyroid hormone in doses sufficient to suppress thyroid-stimulating hormone, since studies have shown a decreased incidence of recurrence.

I-131:

- Studies have shown that a postoperative course of therapeutic (ablative) doses of I-131 results in a decreased recurrence rate in papillary and follicular carcinomas. It should be given in addition to exogenous thyroid hormone.[67]

Stage III Papillary Thyroid Cancer

Standard treatment options:

- Total thyroidectomy plus removal of involved lymph nodes.

- I-131 ablation following total thyroidectomy if the tumor demonstrates uptake of this isotope.[68]

- External-beam irradiation if I-131 uptake is minimal.

---

[67] Beierwaltes WH, Rabbani R, Dmuchowski C, et al.: An analysis of "Ablation of Thyroid Remnants" with I-131 in 511 patients from 1947-1984: experience at University of Michigan. Journal of Nuclear Medicine 25(12): 1287-1293, 1984.

[68] Beierwaltes WH, Rabbani R, Dmuchowski C, et al.: An analysis of "Ablation of Thyroid Remnants" with I-131 in 511 patients from 1947-1984: experience at University of Michigan. Journal of Nuclear Medicine 25(12): 1287-1293, 1984.

160 Thyroid Cancer

Stage III Follicular Thyroid Cancer

Standard treatment options:

- Total thyroidectomy plus removal of involved lymph nodes or other sites of extrathyroid disease.

- I-131 ablation following total thyroidectomy if the tumor demonstrates uptake of this isotope.[69]

- External-beam irradiation if I-131 uptake is minimal.[70]

Stage IV Papillary Thyroid Cancer

The most common sites of metastases are lymph nodes, lung, and bone. Treatment of lymph node metastases alone is often curative. Treatment of distant metastases is usually not curative but may produce significant palliation.

Standard treatment options for distant metastases:

- I-131: Metastases which demonstrate uptake of this isotope may be ablated by therapeutic doses of I-131.

- External-beam irradiation for patients with localized lesions that are unresponsive to I-131.[71]

- Thyroid-stimulating hormone suppression with T-4 is also effective in many of the non I-131 sensitive lesions.

- Patients unresponsive to I-131 should also be considered candidates for investigative protocols testing new approaches to this disease.

Treatment options under clinical evaluation:

- Clinical trials evaluating new treatment approaches to this disease should also be considered for these patients. Chemotherapy has been reported to produce occasional complete responses of long duration.[72] Information

---

[69] Beierwaltes WH, Rabbani R, Dmuchowski C, et al.: An analysis of "Ablation of Thyroid Remnants" with I-131 in 511 patients from 1947-1984: experience at University of Michigan. Journal of Nuclear Medicine 25(12): 1287-1293, 1984.
[70] Simpson WJ, Carruthers JS: The role of external radiation in the management of papillary and follicular thyroid cancer. American Journal of Surgery 136(4): 457-460, 1978.
[71] Simpson WJ, Carruthers JS: The role of external radiation in the management of papillary and follicular thyroid cancer. American Journal of Surgery 136(4): 457-460, 1978.
[72] Gottlieb JA, Hill CS, Ibanez ML, et al.: Chemotherapy of thyroid cancer: an evaluation of experience with 37 patients. Cancer 30(3): 848-853, 1972.

about ongoing clinical trials is available from the NCI (**http://cancer.gov/clinical_trials**).

Stage IV Follicular Thyroid Cancer

Treatment of distant metastases is usually not curative but may produce significant palliation.

Standard treatment options for distant metastases:

- I-131: Metastases which demonstrate uptake of this isotope may be ablated by therapeutic doses of I-131.

- External-beam irradiation for patients with localized lesions that are unresponsive to I-131.[73]

- TSH suppression with T-4 is also effective in many of the non I-131 sensitive lesions.

- Patients unresponsive to I-131 should also be considered candidates for investigative protocols testing new approaches to this disease.

Treatment options under clinical evaluation:

- Clinical trials evaluating new treatment approaches to this disease should also be considered for these patients. Chemotherapy has been reported to produce occasional complete responses of long duration.[74] Information about ongoing clinical trials is available from the NCI (**http://cancer.gov/clinical_trials**).

Harada T, Nishikawa Y, Suzuki T, et al.: Bleomycin treatment for cancer of the thyroid. American Journal of Surgery 122(1): 53-57, 1971.
Shimaoka K, Schoenfeld DA, DeWys WD, et al.: A randomized trial of doxorubicin versus doxorubicin plus cisplatin in patients with advanced thyroid carcinoma. Cancer 56(9): 2155-2160, 1985.
[73] Simpson WJ, Carruthers JS: The role of external radiation in the management of papillary and follicular thyroid cancer. American Journal of Surgery 136(4): 457-460, 1978.
[74] Gottlieb JA, Hill CS, Ibanez ML, et al.: Chemotherapy of thyroid cancer: an evaluation of experience with 37 patients. Cancer 30(3): 848-853, 1972.
Harada T, Nishikawa Y, Suzuki T, et al.: Bleomycin treatment for cancer of the thyroid. American Journal of Surgery 122(1): 53-57, 1971.
Shimaoka K, Schoenfeld DA, DeWys WD, et al.: A randomized trial of doxorubicin versus doxorubicin plus cisplatin in patients with advanced thyroid carcinoma. Cancer 56(9): 2155-2160, 1985.

Medullary Thyroid Cancer

Medullary thyroid cancer (MTC) comprises 5% to 10% of all thyroid cancers. These tumors usually present as a mass in the neck or thyroid, often associated with lymphadenopathy,[75] or they may be diagnosed through screening family members. MTC can also be diagnosed by fine-needle aspiration biopsy. Cytology typically reveals hypercellular tumors with spindle-shaped cells and poor adhesion.[76] Approximately 25% of reported cases of MTC are familial. Familial MTC syndromes include multiple endocrine neoplasia (MEN) 2A, which is the most common, MEN 2B, and familial non-MEN syndromes. Any patient with a familial variant should be screened for other associated endocrine tumors, particularly parathyroid hyperplasia and pheochromocytoma. MTC can secrete calcitonin and other peptide substances. Determining the level of calcitonin is useful for diagnostic purposes and for following the results of treatment. The overall survival of patients with MTC is 65% at 10 years. Poor prognostic factors include advanced age, advanced stage, prior neck surgery, and associated-MEN 2B.[77]

Family members should be screened for calcitonin elevation and/or for the RET proto-oncogene mutation to identify other individuals at risk for developing familial MTC. All patients with MTC (whether familial or sporadic) should be tested for RET mutations, and if they are positive, then family members should also be tested. Whereas modest elevation of calcitonin may lead to a false-positive diagnosis of medullary carcinoma, DNA testing for the RET mutation is the optimal approach. Family members who are gene carriers should undergo prophylactic thyroidectomy at an early age.[78]

---

[75] Soh EY, Clark OH: Surgical considerations and approach to thyroid cancer. Endocrinology and Metabolism Clinics of North America 25(1): 115-139, 1996.
[76] Giuffrida D, Gharib H: Current diagnosis and management of medullary thyroid carcinoma. Annals of Oncology 9(7): 695-701, 1998.
[77] Giuffrida D, Gharib H: Current diagnosis and management of medullary thyroid carcinoma. Annals of Oncology 9(7): 695-701, 1998.
Saad MF, Ordonez NG, Rashid RK, et al.: Medullary carcinoma of the thyroid: a study of the clinical features and prognostic factors in 161 patients. Medicine 63(6); 319-342, 1984.
Bergholm U, Bergstrom R, Ekbom A: Long term follow-up of patients with medullary carcinoma of the thyroid. Cancer 79(1): 132-138, 1997.
[78] Lips CJ, Landsvater RM, Hoppener JW, et al.: Clinical screening as compared with DNA analysis in families with multiple endocrine neoplasia type 2A. New England Journal of Medicine 331(13): 828-835, 1994.
Decker RA, Peacock ML, Borst MJ, et al.: Progress in genetic screening of multiple endocrine neoplasia type 2A: is calcitonin testing obsolete? Surgery 118(2): 257-264, 1995.

Patients with medullary thyroid cancer should be treated with a total thyroidectomy, unless there is evidence of distant metastasis. In patients with clinically palpable medullary carcinoma of the thyroid, the incidence of microscopically positive nodes is over 75%; routine central and bilateral modified neck dissections have been recommended.[79] When cancer is confined to the thyroid gland, the prognosis is excellent.

Radioactive iodine has no place in the treatment of patients with MTC. External radiation therapy has been used for palliation of locally recurrent tumors, without evidence that it provides any survival advantage.[80]

Palliative chemotherapy has been reported to produce occasional responses in patients with metastatic disease.[81] No single drug regimen can be considered standard. Some patients with distant metastases will experience prolonged survival, and can be managed expectantly until they become symptomatic.

Information about ongoing clinical trials is available from the NCI (**http://cancer.gov/clinical_trials**).

Anaplastic Thyroid Cancer

Standard treatment options:

- Surgery: Tracheostomy is frequently necessary. If the disease remains in the local area, which is indeed rare, total thyroidectomy is warranted to reduce symptoms caused by the tumor mass.[82]

---

[79] Moley JF, DeBenedetti MK: Patterns of nodal metastases in palable medullary thyroid carcinoma: recommendations for extent of node dissection. Annals of Surgery 229(6): 880-888, 1999.

[80] Brierley JD, Tsang RW: External radiation therapy in the treatment of thyroid malignancy. Endocrinology and Metabolism Clinics of North America 25(1): 141-157, 1996.

[81] Shimaoka K, Schoenfeld DA, DeWys WD, et al.: A randomized trial of doxorubicin versus doxorubicin plus cisplatin in patients with advanced thyroid carcinoma. Cancer 56(9): 2155-2160, 1985.

De Besi P, Busnardo B, Toso S, et al.: Combined chemotherapy with bleomycin, adriamycin, and platinum in advanced thyroid cancer. Journal of Endocrinological Investigation 14(6): 475-480, 1991.

Wu LT, Averbuch SD, Ball DW, et al.: Treatment of advanced medullary thyroid carcinoma with a combination of cyclophosphamide, vincristine, and dacarbazine. Cancer 73(2): 432-436, 1994.

Orlandi F, Caraci P, Berruti A, et al.: Chemotherapy with dacarbazine and 5-fluorouracil in advanced medullary thyroid cancer. Annals of Oncology 5(8): 763-765, 1994.

[82] Goldman JM, Goren EN, Cohen MH, et al.: Anaplastic thyroid carcinoma: long-term survival after radical surgery. Journal of Surgical Oncology 14(4): 389-394, 1980.

- Radiation therapy: External beam radiation therapy may be employed in those patients who are not surgical candidates or whose tumor cannot be surgically excised.

- Chemotherapy: Anaplastic thyroid cancer is not responsive to I-131 therapy; treatment with single anticancer drugs has been reported to produce partial remissions in some patients. Approximately 30% of patients achieve partial remission with doxorubicin.[83] The combination of doxorubicin plus cisplatin appears to be more active than doxorubicin alone and has been reported to produce more complete responses.[84]

Treatment options under clinical evaluation:

- The combination of chemotherapy plus irradiation in patients following complete resection may provide prolonged survival, but has not been compared to any one modality alone.[85] Clinical trials evaluating new treatment approaches for this disease should also be considered. Information about ongoing clinical trials is available from the NCI (**http://cancer.gov/clinical_trials**).

Recurrent Thyroid Cancer

Patients treated for differentiated thyroid cancer should be followed carefully with physical examinations, thyroglobulin levels, and radiologic studies based on individual risk for recurrent disease.[86] Approximately 10% to 30% of patients felt to be disease-free after initial treatment will develop recurrence and/or metastases. Of patients who recur, approximately 80% recur with disease in the neck alone and 20% with distant metastases. The most common site of distant metastasis is the lung. In a single series of 289 patients who developed recurrences after initial surgery, 16% died of cancer

---

Aldinger KA, Samaan NA, Ibanez ML, et al.: Anaplastic carcinoma of the thyroid: a review of 84 cases of spindle and giant cell carcinoma of the thyroid. Cancer 41(6): 2267-2275, 1978.
[83] Fraker DL, Skarulis M, Livolsi V: Thyroid tumors. In: DeVita VT Jr, Hellman S, Rosenberg SA, eds.: Cancer: Principles and Practice of Oncology. Philadelphia, Pa: Lippincott-Raven Publishers, 5th ed., 1997, pp 1629-1652.
[84] Shimaoka K, Schoenfeld DA, DeWys WD, et al.: A randomized trial of doxorubicin versus doxorubicin plus cisplatin in patients with advanced thyroid carcinoma. Cancer 56(9): 2155-2160, 1985.
[85] Haigh PI, Ituarte PH, Wu HS, et al.: Completely resected anaplastic thyroid carcinoma combined with adjuvant chemotherapy and irradiation is associated with prolonged survival. Cancer 91(12): 2335-2342, 2001.
[86] Ross DS: Long-term management of differentiated thyroid cancer. Endocrinology and Metabolism Clinics of North America 19(3): 719-739, 1990.

at a median time of 5 years following recurrence.[87] The prognosis for patients with clinically detectable recurrences is generally poor, regardless of cell type.[88] However, those patients who recur with local or regional tumor detected only by I-131 scan have a better prognosis.[89] The selection of further treatment depends on many factors, including cell type, uptake of I-131, prior treatment, site of recurrence, and individual patient considerations. Surgery with or without I-131 ablation can be useful in controlling local recurrences, regional node metastases, or occasionally metastases at other localized sites. Approximately half of the patients operated on for recurrent tumor can be rendered free of disease with a second operation.[90] Local and regional recurrences detected by I-131 scan and not clinically apparent can be treated with I-131 ablation and have an excellent prognosis.[91]

Up to 25% of recurrences and metastases from well-differentiated thyroid cancer may not show I-131 uptake. For these patients, other imaging techniques shown to be of value include imaging with thallium-201, magnetic resonance imaging, and pentavalent dimercaptosuccinic acid.[92] When recurrent disease does not concentrate I-131, external-beam or intraoperative radiation therapy can be useful in controlling symptoms related to local tumor recurrences.[93] Systemic chemotherapy can be considered. Chemotherapy has been reported to produce occasional objective responses, usually of short duration.[94] Clinical trials evaluating new treatment approaches should also be considered. Information about ongoing clinical trials is available from the NCI (**http://cancer.gov/clinical_trials**).

---

[87] Mazzaferri EL, Jhiang SM: Long-term impact of initial surgical and medical therapy on papillary and follicular thyroid cancer. American Journal of Medicine 97: 418-428, 1994.

[88] Goretzki PE, Simon D, Frilling A, et al.: Surgical reintervention for differentiated thyroid cancer. British Journal of Surgery 80(8): 1009-1012, 1993.

[89] De Besi P, Busnardo B, Toso S, et al.: Combined chemotherapy with bleomycin, adriamycin, and platinum in advanced thyroid cancer. Journal of Endocrinological Investigation 14(6): 475-480, 1991.

[90] Goretzki PE, Simon D, Frilling A, et al.: Surgical reintervention for differentiated thyroid cancer. British Journal of Surgery 80(8): 1009-1012, 1993.

[91] Coburn M, Teates D, Wanebo HJ: Recurrent thyroid cancer: role of surgery versus radioactive iodine (I131). Annals of Surgery 219(6): 587-595, 1994.

[92] Mallin WH, Elgazzar AH, Maxon HR: Imaging modalities in the follow-up of non-Iodine avid thyroid carcinoma. American Journal of Otolaryngology 15(6): 417-422, 1994.

[93] Vikram B, Strong EW, Shah JP, et al.: Intraoperative radiotherapy in patients with recurrent head and neck cancer. American Journal of Surgery 150(4): 485-487, 1985.

[94] De Besi P, Busnardo B, Toso S, et al.: Combined chemotherapy with bleomycin, adriamycin, and platinum in advanced thyroid cancer. Journal of Endocrinological Investigation 14(6): 475-480, 1991.

Shimaoka K, Schoenfeld DA, DeWys WD, et al.: A randomized trial of doxorubicin versus doxorubicin plus cisplatin in patients with advanced thyroid carcinoma. Cancer 56(9): 2155-2160, 1985.

NIH Databases

In addition to the various Institutes of Health that publish professional guidelines, the NIH has designed a number of databases for professionals.[95] Physician-oriented resources provide a wide variety of information related to the biomedical and health sciences, both past and present. The format of these resources varies. Searchable databases, bibliographic citations, full text articles (when available), archival collections, and images are all available. The following are referenced by the National Library of Medicine:[96]

- **Bioethics:** Access to published literature on the ethical, legal and public policy issues surrounding healthcare and biomedical research. This information is provided in conjunction with the Kennedy Institute of Ethics located at Georgetown University, Washington, D.C.: **http://www.nlm.nih.gov/databases/databases_bioethics.html**

- **HIV/AIDS Resources:** Describes various links and databases dedicated to HIV/AIDS research: **http://www.nlm.nih.gov/pubs/factsheets/aidsinfs.html**

- **NLM Online Exhibitions:** Describes "Exhibitions in the History of Medicine": **http://www.nlm.nih.gov/exhibition/exhibition.html**. Additional resources for historical scholarship in medicine: **http://www.nlm.nih.gov/hmd/hmd.html**

- **Biotechnology Information:** Access to public databases. The National Center for Biotechnology Information conducts research in computational biology, develops software tools for analyzing genome data, and disseminates biomedical information for the better understanding of molecular processes affecting human health and disease: **http://www.ncbi.nlm.nih.gov/**

- **Population Information:** The National Library of Medicine provides access to worldwide coverage of population, family planning, and related health issues, including family planning technology and programs, fertility, and population law and policy: **http://www.nlm.nih.gov/databases/databases_population.html**

- **Cancer Information:** Access to caner-oriented databases: **http://www.nlm.nih.gov/databases/databases_cancer.html**

---

[95] Remember, for the general public, the National Library of Medicine recommends the databases referenced in MEDLINE*plus* (**http://medlineplus.gov/** or **http://www.nlm.nih.gov/medlineplus/databases.html**).

[96] See **http://www.nlm.nih.gov/databases/databases.html**.

- **Profiles in Science:** Offering the archival collections of prominent twentieth-century biomedical scientists to the public through modern digital technology: **http://www.profiles.nlm.nih.gov/**

- **Chemical Information:** Provides links to various chemical databases and references: **http://sis.nlm.nih.gov/Chem/ChemMain.html**

- **Clinical Alerts:** Reports the release of findings from the NIH-funded clinical trials where such release could significantly affect morbidity and mortality: **http://www.nlm.nih.gov/databases/alerts/clinical_alerts.html**

- **Space Life Sciences:** Provides links and information to space-based research (including NASA):
http://www.nlm.nih.gov/databases/databases_space.html

- **MEDLINE:** Bibliographic database covering the fields of medicine, nursing, dentistry, veterinary medicine, the healthcare system, and the pre-clinical sciences:
http://www.nlm.nih.gov/databases/databases_medline.html

- **Toxicology and Environmental Health Information (TOXNET):** Databases covering toxicology and environmental health:
http://sis.nlm.nih.gov/Tox/ToxMain.html

- **Visible Human Interface:** Anatomically detailed, three-dimensional representations of normal male and female human bodies:
http://www.nlm.nih.gov/research/visible/visible_human.html

While all of the above references may be of interest to physicians who study and treat thyroid cancer, the following are particularly noteworthy.

The Combined Health Information Database

A comprehensive source of information on clinical guidelines written for professionals is the Combined Health Information Database. You will need to limit your search to "Brochure/Pamphlet," "Fact Sheet," or "Information Package" and thyroid cancer using the "Detailed Search" option. Go directly to the following hyperlink: **http://chid.nih.gov/detail/detail.html**. To find associations, use the drop boxes at the bottom of the search page where "You may refine your search by." For the publication date, select "All Years," select your preferred language, and the format option "Fact Sheet." By making these selections and typing "thyroid cancer" (or synonyms) into the "For these words:" box above, you will only receive results on fact sheets dealing with thyroid cancer. The following is a sample result:

- **Report on Cancer in Wyoming, 1999**

    Source: Wyoming Cancer Surveillance Program, Wyoming Department of Health, 43 p., 1999.

    Contact: Wyoming Cancer Surveillance Program, Wyoming Department of Health, Hathaway Building, Cheyenne, WY 82002.

    Summary: This report summarizes and tabulates statistics on the occurrence of cancer among Wyoming residents in 1999. The information was extracted from data collected by the Wyoming Cancer Surveillance Program (WCSP). It presents summary statistics on all cancer sites combined and the 16 most reported sites in 1999: (1) Bladder cancer, (2) brain cancer, (3) female breast cancer, (4) colon cancer, (5) corpus uteri cancer, (6) kidney/renal pelvis cancer, (7) leukemia, (8) lung cancer, (9) melanoma (of the skin), (10) nonHodgkin's lymphoma, (11) ovarian cancer, (12) pancreatic cancer, (13) prostate cancer, (14) rectal cancer, (15) stomach cancer, and (16) thyroid cancer. The report also summarizes (1) WCSP research activities initiated in 1998, (2) WCSP research activities initiated in 1997 that are ongoing, and (3) the methodology used by the WCSP in collecting the information.

- **Report on Cancer in Wyoming, 1998**

    Source: Wyoming Cancer Surveillance Program, Wyoming Department of Health, 42 p., 1998.

    Contact: Wyoming Cancer Surveillance Program, Wyoming Department of Health, Hathaway Building, Cheyenne, WY 82009.

    Summary: This report summarizes and tabulates statistics on the occurrence of cancer in Wyoming residents in 1998. The information was extracted from data collected by the Wyoming Cancer Surveillance Program (WCSP). Summary statistics are presented for all cancers combined and the 16 most frequent sites reported in 1998: (1) Bladder cancer, (2) brain cancer, (3) female breast cancer, (4) colon cancer, (5) corpus uteri cancer, (6) kidney/renal pelvis cancer, (7) leukemia, (8) lung cancer, (9) melanoma (of the skin), (10) nonHodgkin's lymphoma, (11) ovarian cancer, (12) pancreatic cancer, (13) prostate cancer, (14) rectal cancer, (15) stomach cancer, and (16) thyroid cancer. The report also summarizes the methodology used by the WCSP in collecting the data.

The NLM Gateway[97]

The NLM (National Library of Medicine) Gateway is a Web-based system that lets users search simultaneously in multiple retrieval systems at the U.S. National Library of Medicine (NLM). It allows users of NLM services to initiate searches from one Web interface, providing "one-stop searching" for many of NLM's information resources or databases.[98] One target audience for the Gateway is the Internet user who is new to NLM's online resources and does not know what information is available or how best to search for it. This audience may include physicians and other healthcare providers, researchers, librarians, students, and, increasingly, patients, their families, and the public.[99] To use the NLM Gateway, simply go to the search site at **http://gateway.nlm.nih.gov/gw/Cmd**. Type "thyroid cancer" (or synonyms) into the search box and click "Search." The results will be presented in a tabular form, indicating the number of references in each database category.

Results Summary

Category	Items Found
Journal Articles	350750
Books / Periodicals / Audio Visual	2586
Consumer Health	294
Meeting Abstracts	2575
Other Collections	87
Total	356292

---

[97] Adapted from NLM: **http://gateway.nlm.nih.gov/gw/Cmd?Overview.x**.
[98] The NLM Gateway is currently being developed by the Lister Hill National Center for Biomedical Communications (LHNCBC) at the National Library of Medicine (NLM) of the National Institutes of Health (NIH).
[99] Other users may find the Gateway useful for an overall search of NLM's information resources. Some searchers may locate what they need immediately, while others will utilize the Gateway as an adjunct tool to other NLM search services such as PubMed® and MEDLINEplus®. The Gateway connects users with multiple NLM retrieval systems while also providing a search interface for its own collections. These collections include various types of information that do not logically belong in PubMed, LOCATORplus, or other established NLM retrieval systems (e.g., meeting announcements and pre-1966 journal citations). The Gateway will provide access to the information found in an increasing number of NLM retrieval systems in several phases.

HSTAT[100]

HSTAT is a free, Web-based resource that provides access to full-text documents used in healthcare decision-making.[101] HSTAT's audience includes healthcare providers, health service researchers, policy makers, insurance companies, consumers, and the information professionals who serve these groups. HSTAT provides access to a wide variety of publications, including clinical practice guidelines, quick-reference guides for clinicians, consumer health brochures, evidence reports and technology assessments from the Agency for Healthcare Research and Quality (AHRQ), as well as AHRQ's Put Prevention Into Practice.[102] Simply search by "thyroid cancer" (or synonyms) at the following Web site: **http://text.nlm.nih.gov**.

Coffee Break: Tutorials for Biologists[103]

Some patients may wish to have access to a general healthcare site that takes a scientific view of the news and covers recent breakthroughs in biology that may one day assist physicians in developing treatments. To this end, we recommend "Coffee Break," a collection of short reports on recent biological discoveries. Each report incorporates interactive tutorials that demonstrate how bioinformatics tools are used as a part of the research process. Currently, all Coffee Breaks are written by NCBI staff.[104] Each report is about 400 words and is usually based on a discovery reported in one or more articles from recently published, peer-reviewed literature.[105] This site has

---

[100] Adapted from HSTAT: **http://www.nlm.nih.gov/pubs/factsheets/hstat.html**.
[101] The HSTAT URL is **http://hstat.nlm.nih.gov/**.
[102] Other important documents in HSTAT include: the National Institutes of Health (NIH) Consensus Conference Reports and Technology Assessment Reports; the HIV/AIDS Treatment Information Service (ATIS) resource documents; the Substance Abuse and Mental Health Services Administration's Center for Substance Abuse Treatment (SAMHSA/CSAT) Treatment Improvement Protocols (TIP) and Center for Substance Abuse Prevention (SAMHSA/CSAP) Prevention Enhancement Protocols System (PEPS); the Public Health Service (PHS) Preventive Services Task Force's *Guide to Clinical Preventive Services*; the independent, nonfederal Task Force on Community Services *Guide to Community Preventive Services*; and the Health Technology Advisory Committee (HTAC) of the Minnesota Health Care Commission (MHCC) health technology evaluations.
[103] Adapted from **http://www.ncbi.nlm.nih.gov/Coffeebreak/Archive/FAQ.html**.
[104] The figure that accompanies each article is frequently supplied by an expert external to NCBI, in which case the source of the figure is cited. The result is an interactive tutorial that tells a biological story.
[105] After a brief introduction that sets the work described into a broader context, the report focuses on how a molecular understanding can provide explanations of observed biology and lead to therapies for diseases. Each vignette is accompanied by a figure and hypertext links that lead to a series of pages that interactively show how NCBI tools and resources are used in the research process.

new articles every few weeks, so it can be considered an online magazine of sorts, and intended for general background information. You can access the Coffee Break Web site at the following hyperlink: **http://www.ncbi.nlm.nih.gov/Coffeebreak/**.

Other Commercial Databases

In addition to resources maintained by official agencies, other databases exist that are commercial ventures addressing medical professionals. Here are a few examples that may interest you:

- **CliniWeb International:** Index and table of contents to selected clinical information on the Internet; see **http://www.ohsu.edu/cliniweb/**.

- **Image Engine:** Multimedia electronic medical record system that integrates a wide range of digitized clinical images with textual data stored in the University of Pittsburgh Medical Center's MARS electronic medical record system; see the following Web site: **http://www.cml.upmc.edu/cml/imageengine/imageEngine.html**.

- **Medical World Search:** Searches full text from thousands of selected medical sites on the Internet; see **http://www.mwsearch.com/**.

- **MedWeaver:** Prototype system that allows users to search differential diagnoses for any list of signs and symptoms, to search medical literature, and to explore relevant Web sites; see **http://www.med.virginia.edu/~wmd4n/medweaver.html**.

- **Metaphrase:** Middleware component intended for use by both caregivers and medical records personnel. It converts the informal language generally used by caregivers into terms from formal, controlled vocabularies; see the following Web site: **http://www.lexical.com/Metaphrase.html**.

The Genome Project and Thyroid Cancer

With all the discussion in the press about the Human Genome Project, it is only natural that physicians, researchers, and patients want to know about how human genes relate to thyroid cancer. In the following section, we will discuss databases and references used by physicians and scientists who work in this area.

Online Mendelian Inheritance in Man (OMIM)

The Online Mendelian Inheritance in Man (OMIM) database is a catalog of human genes and genetic disorders authored and edited by Dr. Victor A. McKusick and his colleagues at Johns Hopkins and elsewhere. OMIM was developed for the World Wide Web by the National Center for Biotechnology Information (NCBI).[106] The database contains textual information, pictures, and reference information. It also contains copious links to NCBI's Entrez database of MEDLINE articles and sequence information.

To search the database, go to **http://www.ncbi.nlm.nih.gov/Omim/searchomim.html**. Type "thyroid cancer" (or synonyms) in the search box, and click "Submit Search." If too many results appear, you can narrow the search by adding the word "clinical." Each report will have additional links to related research and databases. By following these links, especially the link titled "Database Links," you will be exposed to numerous specialized databases that are largely used by the scientific community. These databases are overly technical and seldom used by the general public, but offer an abundance of information. The following is an example of the results you can obtain from the OMIM for thyroid cancer:

- **Achaete-scute Complex, Drosophila, Homolog-like 1**
  Web site: http://www.ncbi.nlm.nih.gov/htbin-post/Omim/dispmim?100790

- **Adenomatous Polyposis of the Colon**
  Web site: http://www.ncbi.nlm.nih.gov/htbin-post/Omim/dispmim?175100

- **Adrenocortical Carcinoma, Hereditary**
  Web site: http://www.ncbi.nlm.nih.gov/htbin-post/Omim/dispmim?202300

- **A-kinase Anchor Protein 13**
  Web site: http://www.ncbi.nlm.nih.gov/htbin-post/Omim/dispmim?604686

---

[106] Adapted from **http://www.ncbi.nlm.nih.gov/**. Established in 1988 as a national resource for molecular biology information, NCBI creates public databases, conducts research in computational biology, develops software tools for analyzing genome data, and disseminates biomedical information--all for the better understanding of molecular processes affecting human health and disease.

- **Alagille Syndrome**
  Web site: http://www.ncbi.nlm.nih.gov/htbin-post/Omim/dispmim?118450

- **Albumin**
  Web site: http://www.ncbi.nlm.nih.gov/htbin-post/Omim/dispmim?103600

- **Androgen Receptor**
  Web site: http://www.ncbi.nlm.nih.gov/htbin-post/Omim/dispmim?313700

- **Atp-binding Cassette, Subfamily A, Member 3**
  Web site: http://www.ncbi.nlm.nih.gov/htbin-post/Omim/dispmim?601615

- **Beckwith-wiedemann Syndrome**
  Web site: http://www.ncbi.nlm.nih.gov/htbin-post/Omim/dispmim?130650

- **Birt-hogg-dube Syndrome**
  Web site: http://www.ncbi.nlm.nih.gov/htbin-post/Omim/dispmim?135150

Genes and Disease (NCBI - Map)

The Genes and Disease database is produced by the National Center for Biotechnology Information of the National Library of Medicine at the National Institutes of Health. This Web site categorizes each disorder by the system of the body associated with it. Go to **http://www.ncbi.nlm.nih.gov/disease/**, and browse the system pages to have a full view of important conditions linked to human genes. Since this site is regularly updated, you may wish to re-visit it from time to time. The following systems and associated disorders are addressed:

- **Cancer:** Uncontrolled cell division.
  Examples: Breast And Ovarian Cancer, Burkitt lymphoma, chronic myeloid leukemia, colon cancer, lung cancer, malignant melanoma, multiple endocrine neoplasia, neurofibromatosis, p53 tumor suppressor, pancreatic cancer, prostate cancer, Ras oncogene, RB: retinoblastoma, von Hippel-Lindau syndrome.
  Web site: **http://www.ncbi.nlm.nih.gov/disease/Cancer.html**

Entrez

Entrez is a search and retrieval system that integrates several linked databases at the National Center for Biotechnology Information (NCBI). These databases include nucleotide sequences, protein sequences, macromolecular structures, whole genomes, and MEDLINE through PubMed. Entrez provides access to the following databases:

- **PubMed:** Biomedical literature (PubMed),
  Web site: **http://www.ncbi.nlm.nih.gov/entrez/query.fcgi?db=PubMed**

- **Nucleotide Sequence Database (Genbank):**
  Web site:
  http://www.ncbi.nlm.nih.gov/entrez/query.fcgi?db=Nucleotide

- **Protein Sequence Database:**
  Web site: **http://www.ncbi.nlm.nih.gov/entrez/query.fcgi?db=Protein**

- **Structure:** Three-dimensional macromolecular structures,
  Web site: **http://www.ncbi.nlm.nih.gov/entrez/query.fcgi?db=Structure**

- **Genome:** Complete genome assemblies,
  Web site: **http://www.ncbi.nlm.nih.gov/entrez/query.fcgi?db=Genome**

- **PopSet:** Population study data sets,
  Web site: **http://www.ncbi.nlm.nih.gov/entrez/query.fcgi?db=Popset**

- **OMIM:** Online Mendelian Inheritance in Man,
  Web site: **http://www.ncbi.nlm.nih.gov/entrez/query.fcgi?db=OMIM**

- **Taxonomy:** Organisms in GenBank,
  Web site:
  http://www.ncbi.nlm.nih.gov/entrez/query.fcgi?db=Taxonomy

- **Books:** Online books,
  Web site: **http://www.ncbi.nlm.nih.gov/entrez/query.fcgi?db=books**

- **ProbeSet:** Gene Expression Omnibus (GEO),
  Web site: **http://www.ncbi.nlm.nih.gov/entrez/query.fcgi?db=geo**

- **3D Domains:** Domains from Entrez Structure,
  Web site: **http://www.ncbi.nlm.nih.gov/entrez/query.fcgi?db=geo**

- **NCBI's Protein Sequence Information Survey Results:**
  Web site: **http://www.ncbi.nlm.nih.gov/About/proteinsurvey/**

To access the Entrez system at the National Center for Biotechnology Information, go to **http://www.ncbi.nlm.nih.gov/entrez/**, and then select the database that you would like to search. The databases available are listed in the drop box next to "Search." In the box next to "for," enter "thyroid cancer" (or synonyms) and click "Go."

Jablonski's Multiple Congenital Anomaly/Mental Retardation (MCA/MR) Syndromes Database[107]

This online resource can be quite useful. It has been developed to facilitate the identification and differentiation of syndromic entities. Special attention is given to the type of information that is usually limited or completely omitted in existing reference sources due to space limitations of the printed form.

At the following Web site you can also search across syndromes using an index: **http://www.nlm.nih.gov/mesh/jablonski/syndrome_toc/toc_a.html**. You can search by keywords at this Web site: **http://www.nlm.nih.gov/mesh/jablonski/syndrome_db.html**.

The Genome Database[108]

Established at Johns Hopkins University in Baltimore, Maryland in 1990, the Genome Database (GDB) is the official central repository for genomic mapping data resulting from the Human Genome Initiative. In the spring of 1999, the Bioinformatics Supercomputing Centre (BiSC) at the Hospital for Sick Children in Toronto, Ontario assumed the management of GDB. The Human Genome Initiative is a worldwide research effort focusing on structural analysis of human DNA to determine the location and sequence of the estimated 100,000 human genes. In support of this project, GDB stores and curates data generated by researchers worldwide who are engaged in the mapping effort of the Human Genome Project (HGP). GDB's mission is to provide scientists with an encyclopedia of the human genome which is continually revised and updated to reflect the current state of scientific knowledge. Although GDB has historically focused on gene mapping, its focus will broaden as the Genome Project moves from mapping to sequence, and finally, to functional analysis.

To access the GDB, simply go to the following hyperlink: **http://www.gdb.org/**. Search "All Biological Data" by "Keyword." Type

---

[107] Adapted from the National Library of Medicine: **http://www.nlm.nih.gov/mesh/jablonski/about_syndrome.html**.
[108] Adapted from the Genome Database: **http://gdbwww.gdb.org/gdb/aboutGDB.html#mission**.

"thyroid cancer" (or synonyms) into the search box, and review the results. If more than one word is used in the search box, then separate each one with the word "and" or "or" (using "or" might be useful when using synonyms). This database is extremely technical as it was created for specialists. The articles are the results which are the most accessible to non-professionals and often listed under the heading "Citations." The contact names are also accessible to non-professionals.

Specialized References

The following books are specialized references written for professionals interested in thyroid cancer (sorted alphabetically by title, hyperlinks provide rankings, information, and reviews at Amazon.com):

- **Advanced and Critical Care Oncology Nursing: Managing Primary Complications** by Cynthia C. Chernecky (Editor), et al; Paperback - 736 pages (September 18, 1997), W B Saunders Co; ISBN: 0721668607; http://www.amazon.com/exec/obidos/ASIN/0721668607/icongroupinterna

- **Cancer: Etiology, Diagnosis, and Treatment** by Walter J. Burdette; Paperback - 287 pages, 1st edition (January 15, 1998), McGraw Hill Text; ISBN: 0070089922; http://www.amazon.com/exec/obidos/ASIN/0070089922/icongroupinterna

- **Cancer Management: A Multidisciplinary Approach: Medical, Surgical & Radiation** by Richard Pazdur (Editor), et al; Paperback - 982 pages, 5th edition (June 15, 2001), Publisher Research & Representation, Inc.; ISBN: 1891483080; http://www.amazon.com/exec/obidos/ASIN/1891483080/icongroupinterna

- **Familial Cancer and Prevention: Molecular Epidemiology: A New Strategy Toward Cancer Control** by Joji Utsunomiya (Editor), et al; Hardcover (April 1999), Wiley-Liss; ISBN: 0471249378; http://www.amazon.com/exec/obidos/ASIN/0471249378/icongroupinterna

- **Fundamentals of Cancer Epidemiology** by Philip C. Nasca, Ph.D. (Editor), Pastides Harris, Ph.D., MPH (Editor); Hardcover - 368 pages, 1st edition (February 15, 2001), Aspen Publishers, Inc.; ISBN: 0834217767; http://www.amazon.com/exec/obidos/ASIN/0834217767/icongroupinterna

- **Helping Cancer Patients Cope: A Problem-Solving Approach** by Arthur M. Nezu (Editor), et al; Hardcover - 314 pages (December 15, 1998), American Psychological Association (APA); ISBN: 1557985332; http://www.amazon.com/exec/obidos/ASIN/1557985332/icongroupinterna

- **Quantitative Estimation and Prediction of Human Cancer Risks (Iarc Scientific Publications, 131)** by Suresh H. Moolgavkar (Editor), et al; Paperback (September 1999), Oxford University Press; ISBN: 9283221311; http://www.amazon.com/exec/obidos/ASIN/9283221311/icongroupinterna
- **Textbook of Cancer Epidemiology** by ADAMI, et al; Hardcover - 385 pages, 1st edition (July 15, 2002), Oxford University Press; ISBN: 0195109694; http://www.amazon.com/exec/obidos/ASIN/0195109694/icongroupinterna

Vocabulary Builder

Acne: A disorder of the skin marked by inflammation of oil glands and hair glands. [NIH]

Bilateral: Affecting both the right and left side of body. [NIH]

Carcinosarcoma: A malignant tumor that is a mixture of carcinoma (cancer of epithelial tissue, which is skin and tissue that lines or covers the internal organs) and sarcoma (cancer of connective tissue, such as bone, cartilage, and fat). [NIH]

Cisplatin: An anticancer drug that belongs to the family of drugs called platinum compounds. [NIH]

Corpus: The body of the uterus. [NIH]

Encephalopathy: A disorder of the brain that can be caused by disease, injury, drugs, or chemicals. [NIH]

Exogenous: Developed or originating outside the organism, as exogenous disease. [EU]

Histology: The study of tissues and cells under a microscope. [NIH]

Immunodeficiency: The decreased ability of the body to fight infection and disease. [NIH]

Ipsilateral: Having to do with the same side of the body. [NIH]

Lymphadenopathy: Disease or swelling of the lymph nodes. [NIH]

Malignancy: A cancerous tumor that can invade and destroy nearby tissue and spread to other parts of the body. [NIH]

Metastasize: To spread from one part of the body to another. When cancer cells metastasize and form secondary tumors, the cells in the metastatic tumor are like those in the original (primary) tumor. [NIH]

MRI: Magnetic resonance imaging (mag-NET-ik REZ-o- nans IM-a-jing). A procedure in which a magnet linked to a computer is used to create detailed pictures of areas inside the body. [NIH]

Occult: Obscure; concealed from observation, difficult to understand. [EU]

Papillomavirus: A genus of papovaviridae causing proliferation of the epithelium, which may lead to malignancy. A wide range of animals are infected including humans, chimpanzees, cattle, rabbits, dogs, and horses. [NIH]

Polyposis: The development of numerous polyps (growths that protrude from a mucous membrane). [NIH]

Postoperative: After surgery. [NIH]

Rectal: By or having to do with the rectum. The rectum is the last 8 to 10 inches of the large intestine and ends at the anus. [NIH]

Retrospective: Looking back at events that have already taken place. [NIH]

Sarcoma: A cancer of the bone, cartilage, fat, muscle, blood vessels or other connective or supportive tissue. [NIH]

Symptomatic: Having to do with symptoms, which are signs of a condition or disease. [NIH]

Teratoma: A type of germ cell tumor that may contain several different types of tissue, such as hair, muscle, and bone. Teratomas occur most often in the ovaries in women, the testicles in men, and the tailbone in children. Not all teratomas are malignant. [NIH]

Thymus: An organ that is part of the lymphatic system, in which T lymphocytes grow and multiply. The thymus is in the chest behind the breastbone. [NIH]

Toxoplasmosis: An acute or chronic, widespread disease of animals and humans caused by the obligate intracellular protozoon Toxoplasma gondii, transmitted by oocysts containing the pathogen in the feces of cats (the definitive host), usually by contaminated soil, direct exposure to infected feces, tissue cysts in infected meat, or tachyzoites (proliferating forms) in blood. [EU]

CHAPTER 9. DISSERTATIONS ON THYROID CANCER

Overview

University researchers are active in studying almost all known diseases. The result of research is often published in the form of Doctoral or Master's dissertations. You should understand, therefore, that applied diagnostic procedures and/or therapies can take many years to develop after the thesis that proposed the new technique or approach was written.

In this chapter, we will give you a bibliography on recent dissertations relating to thyroid cancer. You can read about these in more detail using the Internet or your local medical library. We will also provide you with information on how to use the Internet to stay current on dissertations.

Dissertations on Thyroid Cancer

ProQuest Digital Dissertations is the largest archive of academic dissertations available. From this archive, we have compiled the following list covering dissertations devoted to thyroid cancer. You will see that the information provided includes the dissertation's title, its author, and the author's institution. To read more about the following, simply use the Internet address indicated. The following covers recent dissertations dealing with thyroid cancer:

- **Characterization of RET/PTC1 Transgenic-p53 Knockout Mice and Sodium/iodide Symporter Gene Transfer for Prostate Cancer** by La Perle, Krista Marie Dubray; PhD from The Ohio State University, 2002, 122 pages
  http://wwwlib.umi.com/dissertations/fullcit/3049061
- **Searching for Genes Responsible for Papillary Thyroid Carcinoma** by Huang, Ying; PhD from The Ohio State University, 2002, 177 pages
  http://wwwlib.umi.com/dissertations/fullcit/3049041
- **Statistical Considerations in the Analysis of Matched Case-control Studies: with Applications in Nutritional Epidemiology** by Hansson, Lisbeth Maria; PhD from Uppsala Universitet (Sweden), 2001, 33 pages
  http://wwwlib.umi.com/dissertations/fullcit/f257857

Keeping Current

As previously mentioned, an effective way to stay current on dissertations dedicated to thyroid cancer is to use the database called *ProQuest Digital Dissertations* via the Internet, located at the following Web address: **http://wwwlib.umi.com/dissertations.** The site allows you to freely access the last two years of citations and abstracts. Ask your medical librarian if the library has full and unlimited access to this database. From the library, you should be able to do more complete searches than with the limited 2-year access available to the general public.

PART III. APPENDICES

ABOUT PART III

Part III is a collection of appendices on general medical topics which may be of interest to patients with thyroid cancer and related conditions.

APPENDIX A. RESEARCHING YOUR MEDICATIONS

Overview

There are a number of sources available on new or existing medications which could be prescribed to patients with thyroid cancer. While a number of hard copy or CD-Rom resources are available to patients and physicians for research purposes, a more flexible method is to use Internet-based databases. In this chapter, we will begin with a general overview of medications. We will then proceed to outline official recommendations on how you should view your medications. You may also want to research medications that you are currently taking for other conditions as they may interact with medications for thyroid cancer. Research can give you information on the side effects, interactions, and limitations of prescription drugs used in the treatment of thyroid cancer. Broadly speaking, there are two sources of information on approved medications: public sources and private sources. We will emphasize free-to-use public sources.

Your Medications: The Basics[109]

The Agency for Health Care Research and Quality has published extremely useful guidelines on how you can best participate in the medication aspects of thyroid cancer. Taking medicines is not always as simple as swallowing a pill. It can involve many steps and decisions each day. The AHCRQ recommends that patients with thyroid cancer take part in treatment decisions. Do not be afraid to ask questions and talk about your concerns. By taking a moment to ask questions early, you may avoid problems later. Here are some points to cover each time a new medicine is prescribed:

- Ask about all parts of your treatment, including diet changes, exercise, and medicines.
- Ask about the risks and benefits of each medicine or other treatment you might receive.
- Ask how often you or your doctor will check for side effects from a given medication.

Do not hesitate to ask what is important to you about your medicines. You may want a medicine with the fewest side effects, or the fewest doses to take each day. You may care most about cost, or how the medicine might affect how you live or work. Or, you may want the medicine your doctor believes will work the best. Telling your doctor will help him or her select the best treatment for you.

Do not be afraid to "bother" your doctor with your concerns and questions about medications for thyroid cancer. You can also talk to a nurse or a pharmacist. They can help you better understand your treatment plan. Feel free to bring a friend or family member with you when you visit your doctor. Talking over your options with someone you trust can help you make better choices, especially if you are not feeling well. Specifically, ask your doctor the following:

- The name of the medicine and what it is supposed to do.
- How and when to take the medicine, how much to take, and for how long.
- What food, drinks, other medicines, or activities you should avoid while taking the medicine.
- What side effects the medicine may have, and what to do if they occur.
- If you can get a refill, and how often.

---

[109] This section is adapted from AHCRQ: **http://www.ahcpr.gov/consumer/ncpiebro.htm**.

- About any terms or directions you do not understand.
- What to do if you miss a dose.
- If there is written information you can take home (most pharmacies have information sheets on your prescription medicines; some even offer large-print or Spanish versions).

Do not forget to tell your doctor about all the medicines you are currently taking (not just those for thyroid cancer). This includes prescription medicines and the medicines that you buy over the counter. Then your doctor can avoid giving you a new medicine that may not work well with the medications you take now. When talking to your doctor, you may wish to prepare a list of medicines you currently take, the reason you take them, and how you take them. Be sure to include the following information for each:

- Name of medicine
- Reason taken
- Dosage
- Time(s) of day

Also include any over-the-counter medicines, such as:
- Laxatives
- Diet pills
- Vitamins
- Cold medicine
- Aspirin or other pain, headache, or fever medicine
- Cough medicine
- Allergy relief medicine
- Antacids
- Sleeping pills
- Others (include names)

Learning More about Your Medications

Because of historical investments by various organizations and the emergence of the Internet, it has become rather simple to learn about the medications your doctor has recommended for thyroid cancer. One such source is the United States Pharmacopeia. In 1820, eleven physicians met in Washington, D.C. to establish the first compendium of standard drugs for the United States. They called this compendium the "U.S. Pharmacopeia (USP)." Today, the USP is a non-profit organization consisting of 800 volunteer scientists, eleven elected officials, and 400 representatives of state associations and colleges of medicine and pharmacy. The USP is located in Rockville, Maryland, and its home page is located at **www.usp.org**. The USP currently provides standards for over 3,700 medications. The resulting USP DI® Advice for the Patient® can be accessed through the National Library of Medicine of the National Institutes of Health. The database is partially derived from lists of federally approved medications in the Food and Drug Administration's (FDA) Drug Approvals database.[110]

While the FDA database is rather large and difficult to navigate, the Phamacopeia is both user-friendly and free to use. It covers more than 9,000 prescription and over-the-counter medications. To access this database, simply type the following hyperlink into your Web browser: **http://www.nlm.nih.gov/medlineplus/druginformation.html**. To view examples of a given medication (brand names, category, description, preparation, proper use, precautions, side effects, etc.), simply follow the hyperlinks indicated within the United States Pharmacopoeia (USP). It is important to read the disclaimer by the USP (**http://www.nlm.nih.gov/medlineplus/drugdisclaimer.html**) before using the information provided.

Of course, we as editors cannot be certain as to what medications you are taking. Therefore, we have compiled a list of medications associated with the treatment of thyroid cancer. Once again, due to space limitations, we only list a sample of medications and provide hyperlinks to ample documentation (e.g. typical dosage, side effects, drug-interaction risks, etc.). The following drugs have been mentioned in the Pharmacopeia and other sources as being potentially applicable to thyroid cancer:

Bexarotene
- **Systemic - U.S. Brands:** Targretin
  http://www.nlm.nih.gov/medlineplus/druginfo/bexarotenesystemic500095.html

---

[110] Though cumbersome, the FDA database can be freely browsed at the following site: **www.fda.gov/cder/da/da.htm**.

Bleomycin
- **Systemic - U.S. Brands:** Blenoxane
  http://www.nlm.nih.gov/medlineplus/druginfo/bleomycinsystemic202093.html

Calcitonin
- **Nasal-Systemic - U.S. Brands:** Miacalcin
  http://www.nlm.nih.gov/medlineplus/druginfo/calcitoninnasalsystemic203482.html
- **Systemic - U.S. Brands:** Calcimar; Cibacalcin; Miacalcin
  http://www.nlm.nih.gov/medlineplus/druginfo/calcitoninsystemic202106.html

Cisplatin
- **Systemic - U.S. Brands:** Platinol; Platinol-AQ
  http://www.nlm.nih.gov/medlineplus/druginfo/cisplatinsystemic202143.html

Cyclophosphamide
- **Systemic - U.S. Brands:** Cytoxan; Neosar
  http://www.nlm.nih.gov/medlineplus/druginfo/cyclophosphamidesystemic202174.html

Denileukin Diftitox
- **Systemic - U.S. Brands:** Ontak
  http://www.nlm.nih.gov/medlineplus/druginfo/denileukindiftitoxsystemic500010.html

Etoposide
- **Systemic - U.S. Brands:** Etopophos; Toposar; VePesid
  http://www.nlm.nih.gov/medlineplus/druginfo/etoposidesystemic202234.html

Ifosfamide
- **Systemic - U.S. Brands:** IFEX
  http://www.nlm.nih.gov/medlineplus/druginfo/ifosfamidesystemic202293.html

Interferons, Alpha
- **Systemic - U.S. Brands:** Alferon N; Intron A; Roferon-A
  http://www.nlm.nih.gov/medlineplus/druginfo/interferonsalpha systemic202299.html

Iodine
- **Systemic - U.S. Brands:**
  http://www.nlm.nih.gov/medlineplus/druginfo/calcitoninsyste mic202106.html

Leucovorin
- **Systemic - U.S. Brands:** Wellcovorin
  http://www.nlm.nih.gov/medlineplus/druginfo/leucovorinsyste mic202321.html

Methoxsalen
- **Extracorporeal-Systemic - U.S.** Brands: Uvadex
  http://www.nlm.nih.gov/medlineplus/druginfo/methoxsalenext racorporealsyste500002.html
- **Systemic - U.S. Brands:** 8-MOP; Oxsoralen-Ultra
  http://www.nlm.nih.gov/medlineplus/druginfo/methoxsalensys temic202357.html

Rituximab
- **Systemic - U.S. Brands:** Rituxan
  http://www.nlm.nih.gov/medlineplus/druginfo/rituximabsyste mic203423.html

Teniposide
- **Systemic - U.S. Brands:** Vumon
  http://www.nlm.nih.gov/medlineplus/druginfo/teniposidesyste mic203661.html

Thyroid Hormones
- **Systemic - U.S. Brands:** Armour Thyroid; Cytomel; Levo-T; Levothroid; Levoxyl; Synthroid; Thyrar; Thyroid Strong; Thyrolar; Triostat; Westhroid
  http://www.nlm.nih.gov/medlineplus/druginfo/thyroidhormon essystemic202566.html

Vinblastine
- **Systemic - U.S. Brands:** Velban
  http://www.nlm.nih.gov/medlineplus/druginfo/vinblastinesystemic202593.html

Commercial Databases

In addition to the medications listed in the USP above, a number of commercial sites are available by subscription to physicians and their institutions. You may be able to access these sources from your local medical library or your doctor's office.

Reuters Health Drug Database

The Reuters Health Drug Database can be searched by keyword at the hyperlink: **http://www.reutershealth.com/frame2/drug.html**. The following medications are listed in the Reuters' database as associated with thyroid cancer (including those with contraindications):[111]

- **US anti-radiation pill plan inadequate: experts**
  http://www.reutershealth.com/archive/2002/10/11/eline/links/20021011elin016.htm

Mosby's GenRx

Mosby's GenRx database (also available on CD-Rom and book format) covers 45,000 drug products including generics and international brands. It provides prescribing information, drug interactions, and patient information. Information can be obtained at the following hyperlink: **http://www.genrx.com/Mosby/PhyGenRx/group.html**.

Physicians Desk Reference

The Physicians Desk Reference database (also available in CD-Rom and book format) is a full-text drug database. The database is searchable by brand name, generic name or by indication. It features multiple drug interactions reports. Information can be obtained at the following hyperlink: **http://physician.pdr.net/physician/templates/en/acl/psuser_t.htm**.

---

[111] Adapted from *A to Z Drug Facts* by Facts and Comparisons.

Other Web Sites

A number of additional Web sites discuss drug information. As an example, you may like to look at **www.drugs.com** which reproduces the information in the Pharmacopeia as well as commercial information. You may also want to consider the Web site of the Medical Letter, Inc. which allows users to download articles on various drugs and therapeutics for a nominal fee: **http://www.medletter.com/**.

Drug Development and Approval

The following Web sites can be valuable resources when conducting research on the development and approval of new cancer drugs:

- FDA Home Page: Search for drugs currently in development or those which have been recently approved by the FDA.
  http://redir.nci.nih.gov/cgi-bin/redir.pl?section=Cancerinfo&destURI=http://www.fda.gov/

- Cancer Liaison Program: Answers questions from the public about drug approval processes, cancer clinical trials, and access to investigational therapies.
  http://redir.nci.nih.gov/cgi-bin/redir.pl?section=Cancerinfo&destURI=http://www.fda.gov/oashi/cancer/cancer.html

- Center for Drug Evaluation and Research
  http://redir.nci.nih.gov/cgi-bin/redir.pl?section=Cancerinfo&destURI=http://www.fda.gov/cder/

- Drug Approvals by Cancer Indications (Alphabetical List)
  http://redir.nci.nih.gov/cgi-bin/redir.pl?section=Cancerinfo&destURI=http://www.fda.gov/oashi/cancer/cdrugalpha.html

- Drug Approvals by Cancer Indications (Cancer Type)
  http://redir.nci.nih.gov/cgi-bin/redir.pl?section=Cancerinfo&destURI=http://www.fda.gov/oashi/cancer/cdrugind.html

- Electronic Orange Book of Approved Drug Products
  http://redir.nci.nih.gov/cgi-bin/redir.pl?section=Cancerinfo&destURI=http://www.fda.gov/cder/ob/default.htm

- Guidance Documents for Industry: Contains an archive of documents describing FDA policies on specific topics.
  http://redir.nci.nih.gov/cgi-bin/redir.pl?section=Cancerinfo&destURI=http://www.fda.gov/cder/guidance/index.htm

- Industry Collaboration: Provides information to industry on the process for getting new drugs into clinical trials.
  http://ctep.cancer.gov/industry/index.html

- Investigator's Handbook: Provides information to investigators on specific procedures related to clinical trial development.
  http://ctep.cancer.gov/handbook/index.html

- Questions and Answers About NCI's Natural Products Branch: A fact sheet that describes the functions of this branch, which collects and analyzes specimens of plant, marine, and microbial origin for possible anticancer properties.
  http://cis.nci.nih.gov/fact/7_33.htm

Understanding the Approval Process for New Cancer Drugs[112]

Since June 1996, about 80 new cancer-related drugs, or new uses for drugs already on the market, have been approved by the U.S. Food and Drug Administration (FDA), the division of the U.S. Department of Health and Human Services charged with ensuring the safety and effectiveness of new drugs before they can go on the market. (The FDA maintains an annotated online list of drugs approved for use with cancer since 1996.) Some of these drugs treat cancer, some alleviate pain and other symptoms, and, in one case, reduce the risk of invasive cancer in people who are considered high-risk. The FDA relied on the results of clinical trials in making every one of these approvals. Without reliable information about a drug's effects on humans, it would be impossible to approve any drug for widespread use.

When considering a new drug, the FDA faces two challenges:

- First, making sure that the drug is safe and effective before it is made widely available;

- Second, ensuring that drugs which show promise are made available as quickly as possible to the people they can help.

---

[112] Adapted from the NCI: http://www.cancer.gov/clinical_trials/doc_header.aspx?viewid=d94cbfac-e478-4704-9052-d8e8a3372b56.

To deal with these challenges, the FDA maintains a rigorous review process but also has measures in place to make some drugs available in special cases. This aim of this section is to acquaint you with the drug approval process and point you to other resources for learning more about it.

The Role of the Federal Drug Administration (FDA)

Approval is only one step in the drug development process. In fact, the FDA estimates that, on average, it takes eight and a half years to study and test a new drug before it can be approved for the general public. That includes early laboratory and animal testing, as well as the clinical trials that evaluate the drugs in humans. The FDA plays a key role at three main points in this process:

- Determining whether or not a new drug shows enough promise to be given to people in clinical trials

- Once clinical trials begin, deciding whether or not they should continue, based on reports of efficacy and adverse reactions

- When clinical trials are completed, deciding whether or not the drug can be sold to the public and what its label should say about directions for use, side effects, warnings, and the like.

To make these decisions, the FDA must review studies submitted by the drug's sponsor (usually the manufacturer), evaluate any adverse reports from preclinical studies and clinical trials (that is, reports of side effects or complications), and review the adequacy of the chemistry and manufacturing. This process is lengthy, but it is meant to ensure that only beneficial drugs with acceptable side effects will make their way into the hands of the public. At the same time, recent legislative mandates and streamlined procedures within the FDA have accelerated the approval of effective drugs, especially for serious illnesses such as cancer. In addition, specific provisions make some drugs available to patients with special needs even before the approval process is complete.

From Lab to Patient Care

By law, the Food and Drug Administration (FDA) must review all test results for new drugs to ensure that products are safe and effective for specific uses. "Safe" does not mean that the drug is free of possible adverse side effects; rather, it means that the potential benefits have been determined to outweigh any risks. The testing process begins long before the first person takes the drug, with preliminary research and animal testing.

If a drug proves promising in the lab, the drug company or sponsor must apply for FDA approval to test it in clinical trials involving people. For drugs, the application, called an Investigational New Drug (IND) Application, is sent through the Center for Drug Evaluation and Research's (CDER) IND Review Process; for biological agents, the IND is sent to the Center for Biologics Evaluation and Research (CBER). Once the IND is approved by CDER or CBER, clinical trials can begin.

If the drug makes it through the clinical trials process—that is, the studies show that it is superior to current drugs—the manufacturer must submit a New Drug Application (NDA) or (for biological agents) a Biologics License Application (BLA) to the FDA. (Biological agents, such as serums, vaccines, and cloned proteins, are manufactured from substances taken from living humans or animals.) This application must include:

- The exact chemical makeup of the drug or biologic and the mechanisms by which it is effective
- Results of animal studies
- Results of clinical trials
- How the drug or biologic is manufactured, processed, and packaged
- Quality control standards
- Samples of the product in the form(s) in which it is to be administered.

Once the FDA receives the NDA or BLA from the manufacturer or developer, the formal New Drug Application Review Process or Biologics/Product License Application Review Process begins.

For an overview of the entire process from start to finish, see the CDER's visual representation of The New Drug Development Process: Steps from Test Tube to New Drug Application Review, which is available for public viewing at the following Web address: **http://www.fda.gov/cder/handbook/develop.htm**.

Speed versus Safety in the Approval Process

The FDA's current goal is that no more than ten months will pass between the time that a complete application is submitted and the FDA takes action on it. But the process is not always smooth. Sometimes FDA's external advisory panels call for additional research or data. In other cases, the FDA staff asks for more information or revised studies. Some new drug approvals have taken as little as 42 days; other more difficult NDAs have spent years in the approval process.

Setting Priorities

The order in which NDAs are assessed by the FDA is determined by a classification system designed to give priority to drugs with the greatest potential benefits. All drugs that offer significant medical advances over existing therapies for any disease are considered "priority" drugs in the approval process. NDAs for cancer treatment drugs are reviewed for this status primarily by the Division of Oncology Drug Products in the FDA's Center for Drug Evaluation and Research (CDER). For Biologic License Applications (vaccines, blood products, and medicines made from animal products), the Center for Biologics Evaluation and Research (CBER) provides additional regulation and oversight.

Expert Advice

The FDA relies on a system of independent advisory committees, made up of professionals from outside the agency, for expert advice and guidance in making sound decisions about drug approval. Each committee meets as needed to weigh available evidence and assess the safety, effectiveness, and appropriate use of products considered for approval. In addition, these committees provide advice about general criteria for evaluation and scientific issues not related to specific products. The Oncologic Drugs Advisory Committee (ODAC) meets regularly to provide expert advice on cancer-related treatments and preventive drugs.

Each committee is composed of representatives from the research science and medical fields. At least one member on every advisory committee must represent the consumer perspective.

Final Approval

As the FDA looks at all the data submitted and the results of its own review, it applies two benchmark questions to each application for drug approval:

- Do the results of well-controlled studies provide substantial evidence of effectiveness?
- Do the results show the product is safe under the conditions of use in the proposed labeling? In this context, "safe" means that potential benefits have been determined to outweigh any risks.

Continued Vigilance

The FDA's responsibility for new drug treatments does not stop with final approval. The Office of Compliance in the Center for Drug Evaluation and Research (CDER) implements and tracks programs to make sure manufacturers comply with current standards and practice regulations. CDER's Office of Drug Marketing, Advertising, and Communication monitors new drug advertising to make sure it is truthful and complete. At the Center for Biologic Evaluation and Research, biologics are followed with the same vigilance after approval. And through a system called MedWatch, the FDA gets feedback from health professionals and consumers on how the new drugs are working, any adverse reactions, and potential problems in labeling and dosage.

Online FDA Resources

The following information from the FDA should help you better understand the drug approval process:

- Center for Drug Evaluation and Research:
  http://www.fda.gov/cder/handbook
- From Test Tube to Patient: New Drug Development in the U.S. – a special January 1995 issue of the magazine FDA Consumer:
  http://www.fda.gov/fdac/special/newdrug/ndd_toc.html
- Milestones in U.S. Food and Drug Law History:
  http://www.fda.gov/opacom/backgrounders/miles.html
- Drug Approvals for Cancer Indications:
  http://www.fda.gov/oashi/cancer/cdrug.html

Getting Drugs to Patients Who Need Them

Clinical trials provide the most important information used by the FDA in determining whether a new drug shows "substantial evidence of effectiveness," or whether an already-approved drug can be used effectively in new ways (for example, to treat or prevent other types of cancer, or at a different dosage). The FDA must certify that a drug has shown promise in laboratory and animal trials before human testing can begin. The trials process includes three main stages and involves continuous review, which ensures that the sponsor can stop the study early if major problems develop or unexpected levels of treatment benefit are found. As with all clinical trials, benefits and risks must be carefully weighed by the researchers conducting the study and the patients who decide to participate.

Not everyone is eligible to participate in a clinical trial. Some patients do not fit the exact requirements for studies, some have rare forms of cancer for which only a limited number of studies are underway, and others are too ill to participate. Working with the NCI and other sponsors, the FDA has established special conditions under which a patient and his or her physician can apply to receive cancer drugs that have not yet been through the approval process. In the past, these special case applications for new drugs were grouped under the name "compassionate uses." More recently, such uses have expanded to include more patients and more categories of investigational drugs.

Access to Investigational Drugs

The process of new drug development has many parts. In the United States, until a drug has been approved by the FDA, it can generally be obtained only through several mechanisms: enrollment in a clinical trial studying the drug, an expanded access program or special exemption/compassionate use programs. For more information about investigational drugs, see "Questions and Answers: Access to Investigational Drugs" at **http://www.cancer.gov/cancer_information/doc_img.aspx?viewid=74b62d84-e135-451f-9bc9-d54358ede947**.

"Group C" Drugs

In the 1970s, researchers from the NCI became concerned about the lag between the date when an investigational drug was found to have anti-tumor activity and the time that drug became available on the market. Working with the FDA, the NCI established the "Group C" classification to allow access to drugs with reproducible activity. Group C drugs are provided to properly trained physicians who have registered using a special form to assure that their patient qualifies under guideline protocols for the drug. Each Group C drug protocol specifies patient eligibility, reporting methodology, and drug use. Not only does Group C designation (now called Group C/Treatment INDs) speed new drugs to patients who need them most, but the process also allows the NCI to gather important information on the safety as well as activity of the drugs in the settings in which they will be most used after final FDA approval. Drugs are placed in the Group C category by agreement between the FDA and the NCI. Group C drugs are always provided free of charge, and the Health Care Financing Administration provides coverage for care associated with Group C therapy.

Treatment INDs

In 1987, the FDA began authorizing the use of new drugs still in the development process to treat certain seriously ill patients. In these cases, the process is referred to as a treatment investigational new drug application (Treatment IND). Clinical trials of the new drug must already be underway and have demonstrated positive results that are reproducible. The FDA sets guidelines about what constitutes serious and life-threatening illnesses, how much must already be known about a drug's side effects and benefits, and where physicians can obtain the drug for treatment. For many seriously ill patients, the risks associated with taking a not-yet-completely proven drug are outweighed by the possible benefits.

Accelerated Approval

"Accelerated approval" is the short-hand term for the FDA's new review system which, in the 1990s, has been used to ensure rapid approval while at the same time putting new safeguards into place. Accelerated approval is based on "surrogate endpoint" judgments: FDA can grant marketing approval to drugs and treatments that, according to certain indicators, prove they are likely to have beneficial effects on a disease or condition, even before such direct benefits have been shown clinically. Accelerated approval does NOT mean that additional clinical trials are not needed or that FDA stops gathering information about the effects of the drug; a follow-up study is required to demonstrate activity by more conventional endpoints.

Contraindications and Interactions (Hidden Dangers)

Some of the medications mentioned in the previous discussions can be problematic for patients with thyroid cancer--not because they are used in the treatment process, but because of contraindications, or side effects. Medications with contraindications are those that could react with drugs used to treat thyroid cancer or potentially create deleterious side effects in patients with thyroid cancer. You should ask your physician about any contraindications, especially as these might apply to other medications that you may be taking for common ailments.

Drug-drug interactions occur when two or more drugs react with each other. This drug-drug interaction may cause you to experience an unexpected side effect. Drug interactions may make your medications less effective, cause unexpected side effects, or increase the action of a particular drug. Some drug interactions can even be harmful to you.

Be sure to read the label every time you use a nonprescription or prescription drug, and take the time to learn about drug interactions. These precautions may be critical to your health. You can reduce the risk of potentially harmful drug interactions and side effects with a little bit of knowledge and common sense.

Drug labels contain important information about ingredients, uses, warnings, and directions which you should take the time to read and understand. Labels also include warnings about possible drug interactions. Further, drug labels may change as new information becomes available. This is why it's especially important to read the label every time you use a medication. When your doctor prescribes a new drug, discuss all over-the-counter and prescription medications, dietary supplements, vitamins, botanicals, minerals and herbals you take as well as the foods you eat. Ask your pharmacist for the package insert for each prescription drug you take. The package insert provides more information about potential drug interactions.

A Final Warning

At some point, you may hear of alternative medications from friends, relatives, or in the news media. Advertisements may suggest that certain alternative drugs can produce positive results for patients with thyroid cancer. Exercise caution--some of these drugs may have fraudulent claims, and others may actually hurt you. The Food and Drug Administration (FDA) is the official U.S. agency charged with discovering which medications are likely to improve the health of patients with thyroid cancer. The FDA warns patients to watch out for[113]:

- Secret formulas (real scientists share what they know)
- Amazing breakthroughs or miracle cures (real breakthroughs don't happen very often; when they do, real scientists do not call them amazing or miracles)
- Quick, painless, or guaranteed cures
- If it sounds too good to be true, it probably isn't true.

If you have any questions about any kind of medical treatment, the FDA may have an office near you. Look for their number in the blue pages of the phone book. You can also contact the FDA through its toll-free number, 1-888-INFO-FDA (1-888-463-6332), or on the World Wide Web at **www.fda.gov**.

General References

In addition to the resources provided earlier in this chapter, the following general references describe medications (sorted alphabetically by title; hyperlinks provide rankings, information and reviews at Amazon.com):

- **Antifolate Drugs in Cancer Therapy (Cancer Drug Discovery and Development)** by Ann L. Jackman (Editor); Hardcover: 480 pages; (March 1999), Humana Press; ISBN: 0896035964;
  http://www.amazon.com/exec/obidos/ASIN/0896035964/icongroupinterna

- **Consumers Guide to Cancer Drugs** by Gail M. Wilkes, et al; Paperback - 448 pages, 1st edition (January 15, 2000), Jones & Bartlett Publishing; ISBN: 0763711705;
  http://www.amazon.com/exec/obidos/ASIN/0763711705/icongroupinterna

---

[113] This section has been adapted from **http://www.fda.gov/opacom/lowlit/medfraud.html**

- **Patient Education Guide to Oncology Drugs (Book with CD-ROM)** by Gail M. Wilkes, et al; CD-ROM - 447 pages, 1st edition (January 15, 2000), Jones & Bartlett Publishing; ISBN: 076371173X; http://www.amazon.com/exec/obidos/ASIN/076371173X/icongroupinterna
- **The Role of Multiple Intensification in Medical Oncology** by M. S. Aapro (Editor), D. Maraninchi (Editor); Hardcover (June 1998), Springer Verlag; ISBN: 3540635432; http://www.amazon.com/exec/obidos/ASIN/3540635432/icongroupinterna

Vocabulary Builder

The following vocabulary builder gives definitions of words used in this chapter that have not been defined in previous chapters:

Aspirin: A drug that reduces pain, fever, inflammation, and blood clotting. Aspirin belongs to the family of drugs called nonsteroidal anti-inflammatory agents. It is also being studied in cancer prevention. [NIH]

Extracorporeal: Situated or occurring outside the body. [EU]

Ifosfamide: An anticancer drug that belongs to the family of drugs called alkylating agents. [NIH]

Leucovorin: A drug used to protect normal cells from high doses of the anticancer drug methotrexate. It is also used to increase the antitumor effects of fluorouracil and tegafur-uracil, an oral treatment alternative to intravenous fluorouracil. [NIH]

Teniposide: An anticancer drug that is a podophyllotoxin derivative and belongs to the family of drugs called mitotic inhibitors. [NIH]

Thyroid Hormones: Hormones secreted by the thyroid gland. [NIH]

Vinblastine: An anticancer drug that belongs to the family of plant drugs called vinca alkaloids. It is a mitotic inhibitor. [NIH]

APPENDIX B. RESEARCHING ALTERNATIVE MEDICINE

Overview[114]

Research indicates that the use of complementary and alternative therapies is increasing. A large-scale study published in the November 11, 1998, issue of the Journal of the American Medical Association found that CAM use among the general public increased from 34 percent in 1990 to 42 percent in 1997.

Several surveys of CAM use by cancer patients have been conducted with small numbers of patients. One study published in the February 2000 issue of the journal *Cancer* reported that 37 percent of 46 patients with prostate cancer used one or more CAM therapies as part of their cancer treatment. These therapies included herbal remedies, old-time remedies, vitamins, and special diets. A larger study of CAM use in patients with different types of cancer was published in the July 2000 issue of the Journal of Clinical Oncology . That study found that 83 percent of 453 cancer patients had used at least one CAM therapy as part of their cancer treatment. The study included CAM therapies such as special diets, psychotherapy, spiritual practices, and vitamin supplements. When psychotherapy and spiritual practices were excluded, 69 percent of patients had used at least one CAM therapy in their cancer treatment.

In this chapter, we will begin by giving you a broad perspective on complementary and alternative therapies. Next, we will introduce you to official information sources on CAM relating to thyroid cancer. Finally, at the conclusion of this chapter, we will provide a list of readings on thyroid cancer from various authors. We will begin, however, with the National

---

[114] Adapted from the NCI: **http://cis.nci.nih.gov/fact/9_14.htm**.

Center for Complementary and Alternative Medicine's (NCCAM) overview of complementary and alternative medicine.

What Is CAM?[115]

Complementary and alternative medicine (CAM) covers a broad range of healing philosophies, approaches, and therapies. Generally, it is defined as those treatments and healthcare practices which are not taught in medical schools, used in hospitals, or reimbursed by medical insurance companies. Many CAM therapies are termed "holistic," which generally means that the healthcare practitioner considers the whole person, including physical, mental, emotional, and spiritual health. Some of these therapies are also known as "preventive," which means that the practitioner educates and treats the person to prevent health problems from arising, rather than treating symptoms after problems have occurred.

People use CAM treatments and therapies in a variety of ways. Therapies are used alone (often referred to as alternative), in combination with other alternative therapies, or in addition to conventional treatment (sometimes referred to as complementary). Complementary and alternative medicine, or "integrative medicine," includes a broad range of healing philosophies, approaches, and therapies. Some approaches are consistent with physiological principles of Western medicine, while others constitute healing systems with non-Western origins. While some therapies are far outside the realm of accepted Western medical theory and practice, others are becoming established in mainstream medicine.

Complementary and alternative therapies are used in an effort to prevent illness, reduce stress, prevent or reduce side effects and symptoms, or control or cure disease. Some commonly used methods of complementary or alternative therapy include mind/body control interventions such as visualization and relaxation, manual healing including acupressure and massage, homeopathy, vitamins or herbal products, and acupuncture.

Should you wish to explore non-traditional types of treatment, be sure to discuss all issues concerning treatments and therapies with your healthcare provider, whether a physician or practitioner of complementary and alternative medicine. Competent healthcare management requires knowledge of both conventional and alternative therapies you are taking for the practitioner to have a complete picture of your treatment plan.

---

[115] Adapted from the NCCAM: **http://nccam.nih.gov/nccam/fcp/faq/index.html#what-is**.

The decision to use complementary and alternative treatments is an important one. Consider before selecting an alternative therapy, the safety and effectiveness of the therapy or treatment, the expertise and qualifications of the healthcare practitioner, and the quality of delivery. These topics should be considered when selecting any practitioner or therapy.

What Are the Domains of Alternative Medicine?[116]

The list of CAM practices changes continually. The reason being is that these new practices and therapies are often proved to be safe and effective, and therefore become generally accepted as "mainstream" healthcare practices. Today, CAM practices may be grouped within five major domains: (1) alternative medical systems, (2) mind-body interventions, (3) biologically-based treatments, (4) manipulative and body-based methods, and (5) energy therapies. The individual systems and treatments comprising these categories are too numerous to list in this sourcebook. Thus, only limited examples are provided within each.

Alternative Medical Systems

Alternative medical systems involve complete systems of theory and practice that have evolved independent of, and often prior to, conventional biomedical approaches. Many are traditional systems of medicine that are practiced by individual cultures throughout the world, including a number of venerable Asian approaches.

Traditional oriental medicine emphasizes the balance or disturbances of qi (pronounced chi) or vital energy in health and disease, respectively. Traditional oriental medicine consists of a group of techniques and methods including acupuncture, herbal medicine, oriental massage, and qi gong (a form of energy therapy). Acupuncture involves stimulating specific anatomic points in the body for therapeutic purposes, usually by puncturing the skin with a thin needle.

Ayurveda is India's traditional system of medicine. Ayurvedic medicine (meaning "science of life") is a comprehensive system of medicine that places equal emphasis on body, mind, and spirit. Ayurveda strives to restore the innate harmony of the individual. Some of the primary Ayurvedic

---

[116] Adapted from the NCCAM: **http://nccam.nih.gov/nccam/fcp/classify/index.html**

treatments include diet, exercise, meditation, herbs, massage, exposure to sunlight, and controlled breathing.

Other traditional healing systems have been developed by the world's indigenous populations. These populations include Native American, Aboriginal, African, Middle Eastern, Tibetan, and Central and South American cultures. Homeopathy and naturopathy are also examples of complete alternative medicine systems.

Homeopathic medicine is an unconventional Western system that is based on the principle that "like cures like," i.e., that the same substance that in large doses produces the symptoms of an illness, in very minute doses cures it. Homeopathic health practitioners believe that the more dilute the remedy, the greater its potency. Therefore, they use small doses of specially prepared plant extracts and minerals to stimulate the body's defense mechanisms and healing processes in order to treat illness.

Naturopathic medicine is based on the theory that disease is a manifestation of alterations in the processes by which the body naturally heals itself and emphasizes health restoration rather than disease treatment. Naturopathic physicians employ an array of healing practices, including the following: diet and clinical nutrition, homeopathy, acupuncture, herbal medicine, hydrotherapy (the use of water in a range of temperatures and methods of applications), spinal and soft-tissue manipulation, physical therapies (such as those involving electrical currents, ultrasound, and light), therapeutic counseling, and pharmacology.

Mind-Body Interventions

Mind-body interventions employ a variety of techniques designed to facilitate the mind's capacity to affect bodily function and symptoms. Only a select group of mind-body interventions having well-documented theoretical foundations are considered CAM. For example, patient education and cognitive-behavioral approaches are now considered "mainstream." On the other hand, complementary and alternative medicine includes meditation, certain uses of hypnosis, dance, music, and art therapy, as well as prayer and mental healing.

Biological-Based Therapies

This category of CAM includes natural and biological-based practices, interventions, and products, many of which overlap with conventional medicine's use of dietary supplements. This category includes herbal, special dietary, orthomolecular, and individual biological therapies.

Herbal therapy employs an individual herb or a mixture of herbs for healing purposes. An herb is a plant or plant part that produces and contains chemical substances that act upon the body. Special diet therapies, such as those proposed by Drs. Atkins, Ornish, Pritikin, and Weil, are believed to prevent and/or control illness as well as promote health. Orthomolecular therapies aim to treat disease with varying concentrations of chemicals such as magnesium, melatonin, and mega-doses of vitamins. Biological therapies include, for example, the use of laetrile and shark cartilage to treat cancer and the use of bee pollen to treat autoimmune and inflammatory diseases.

Manipulative and Body-Based Methods

This category includes methods that are based on manipulation and/or movement of the body. For example, chiropractors focus on the relationship between structure and function, primarily pertaining to the spine, and how that relationship affects the preservation and restoration of health. Chiropractors use manipulative therapy as an integral treatment tool.

In contrast, osteopaths place particular emphasis on the musculoskeletal system and practice osteopathic manipulation. Osteopaths believe that all of the body's systems work together and that disturbances in one system may have an impact upon function elsewhere in the body. Massage therapists manipulate the soft tissues of the body to normalize those tissues.

Energy Therapies

Energy therapies focus on energy fields originating within the body (biofields) or those from other sources (electromagnetic fields). Biofield therapies are intended to affect energy fields (the existence of which is not yet experimentally proven) that surround and penetrate the human body. Some forms of energy therapy manipulate biofields by applying pressure and/or manipulating the body by placing the hands in or through these fields. Examples include Qi gong, Reiki and Therapeutic Touch.

Qi gong is a component of traditional oriental medicine that combines movement, meditation, and regulation of breathing to enhance the flow of vital energy (qi) in the body, improve blood circulation, and enhance immune function. Reiki, the Japanese word representing Universal Life Energy, is based on the belief that, by channeling spiritual energy through the practitioner, the spirit is healed and, in turn, heals the physical body. Therapeutic Touch is derived from the ancient technique of "laying-on of hands." It is based on the premises that the therapist's healing force affects the patient's recovery and that healing is promoted when the body's energies are in balance. By passing their hands over the patient, these healers identify energy imbalances.

Bioelectromagnetic-based therapies involve the unconventional use of electromagnetic fields to treat illnesses or manage pain. These therapies are often used to treat asthma, cancer, and migraine headaches. Types of electromagnetic fields which are manipulated in these therapies include pulsed fields, magnetic fields, and alternating current or direct current fields.

Research indicates that the use of complementary and alternative therapies is increasing. A large-scale study published in the November 11, 1998, issue of the Journal of the American Medical Association found that CAM use among the general public increased from 34 percent in 1990 to 42 percent in 1997.

Several surveys of CAM use by cancer patients have been conducted with small numbers of patients. One study published in the February 2000 issue of the journal Cancer reported that 37 percent of 46 patients with prostate cancer used one or more CAM therapies as part of their cancer treatment. These therapies included herbal remedies, old-time remedies, vitamins, and special diets. A larger study of CAM use in patients with different types of cancer was published in the July 2000 issue of the Journal of Clinical Oncology . That study found that 83 percent of 453 cancer patients had used at least one CAM therapy as part of their cancer treatment. The study included CAM therapies such as special diets, psychotherapy, spiritual practices, and vitamin supplements. When psychotherapy and spiritual practices were excluded, 69 percent of patients had used at least one CAM therapy in their cancer treatment.

How Are Complementary and Alternative Approaches Evaluated?[117]

It is important that the same scientific evaluation which is used to assess conventional approaches be used to evaluate complementary and alternative therapies. A number of medical centers are evaluating complementary and alternative therapies by developing clinical trials (research studies with people) to test them.

Conventional approaches to cancer treatment have generally been studied for safety and effectiveness through a rigorous scientific process, including clinical trials with large numbers of patients. Often, less is known about the safety and effectiveness of complementary and alternative methods. Some of these complementary and alternative therapies have not undergone rigorous evaluation. Others, once considered unorthodox, are finding a place in cancer treatment—not as cures, but as complementary therapies that may help patients feel better and recover faster. One example is acupuncture. According to a panel of experts at a National Institutes of Health (NIH) Consensus Conference in November 1997, acupuncture has been found to be effective in the management of chemotherapy-associated nausea and vomiting and in controlling pain associated with surgery. Some approaches, such as laetrile, have been studied and found ineffective or potentially harmful.

NCI-Sponsored Clinical Trials in Complementary and Alternative Medicine

The NCI is currently sponsoring several clinical trials (research studies with patients) that study complementary and alternative treatments for cancer. Current trials include enzyme therapy with nutritional support for the treatment of inoperable pancreatic cancer, shark cartilage therapy for the treatment of non-small cell lung cancer, and studies of the effects of diet on prostate and breast cancers. Some of these trials compare alternative therapies with conventional treatments, while others study the effects of complementary approaches used in addition to conventional treatments. Patients who are interested in taking part in these or any clinical trials should talk with their doctor.

More information about clinical trials sponsored by the NCI can be obtained from NCCAM (http://nccam.nih.gov, 1-888-644-6226), OCCAM

---

[117] Adapted from the NCI: **http://cis.nci.nih.gov/fact/9_14.htm**

(http://occam.nci.nih.gov), and the NCI's Cancer Information Service (CIS) (http://cis.nci.nih.gov, 1-800-4-CANCER).

Questions to Ask Your Healthcare Provider about CAM

When considering complementary and alternative therapies, ask your healthcare provider the following questions:

- What benefits can be expected from this therapy?
- What are the risks associated with this therapy?
- Do the known benefits outweigh the risks?
- What side effects can be expected?
- Will the therapy interfere with conventional treatment?
- Is this therapy part of a clinical trial? If so, who is sponsoring the trial?
- Will the therapy be covered by health insurance?
- How can patients and their health care providers learn more about complementary and alternative therapies?

Finding CAM References on Thyroid Cancer

Having read the previous discussion, you may be wondering which complementary or alternative treatments might be appropriate for thyroid cancer. For the remainder of this chapter, we will direct you to a number of official sources which can assist you in researching studies and publications. Some of these articles are rather technical, so some patience may be required.

National Center for Complementary and Alternative Medicine

The National Center for Complementary and Alternative Medicine (NCCAM) of the National Institutes of Health (http://nccam.nih.gov) has created a link to the National Library of Medicine's databases to allow patients to search for articles that specifically relate to thyroid cancer and complementary medicine. To search the database, go to the following Web site: **www.nlm.nih.gov/nccam/camonpubmed.html**. Select "CAM on PubMed." Enter "thyroid cancer" (or synonyms) into the search box. Click "Go." The following references provide information on particular aspects of complementary and alternative medicine (CAM) that are related to thyroid cancer:

- **Adjuvant treatment of thyroid cancer.**
  Author(s): Beauduin M, Hermans J, Majois F.
  Source: Acta Otorhinolaryngol Belg. 1987; 41(5): 944-5. No Abstract Available.
  http://www.ncbi.nlm.nih.gov:80/entrez/query.fcgi?cmd=Retrieve&db=PubMed&list_uids=3454107&dopt=Abstract

- **Assessment of combined radioimmunotherapy and chemotherapy for treatment of medullary thyroid cancer.**
  Author(s): Stein R, Juweid M, Zhang CH, Goldenberg DM.
  Source: Clinical Cancer Research : an Official Journal of the American Association for Cancer Research. 1999 October; 5(10 Suppl): 3199S-3206S.
  http://www.ncbi.nlm.nih.gov:80/entrez/query.fcgi?cmd=Retrieve&db=PubMed&list_uids=10541364&dopt=Abstract

- Chemotherapy for thyroid cancer.
  Author(s): Hoskin PJ, Harmer C.
  Source: Radiotherapy and Oncology : Journal of the European Society for Therapeutic Radiology and Oncology. 1987 November; 10(3): 187-94.
  http://www.ncbi.nlm.nih.gov:80/entrez/query.fcgi?cmd=Retrieve&db=PubMed&list_uids=2448847&dopt=Abstract

- Chemotherapy of thyroid cancer. An evaluation of experience with 37 patients.
  Author(s): Gottlieb JA, Hill CS Jr, Ibanez ML, Clark RL.
  Source: Cancer. 1972 September; 30(3): 848-53. No Abstract Available.
  http://www.ncbi.nlm.nih.gov:80/entrez/query.fcgi?cmd=Retrieve&db=PubMed&list_uids=5075365&dopt=Abstract

- Combination chemotherapy of advanced medullary and differentiated thyroid cancer. Phase II study.
  Author(s): Scherubl H, Raue F, Ziegler R.
  Source: Journal of Cancer Research and Clinical Oncology. 1990; 116(1): 21-3.
  http://www.ncbi.nlm.nih.gov:80/entrez/query.fcgi?cmd=Retrieve&db=PubMed&list_uids=2312602&dopt=Abstract

- Combination chemotherapy of metastatic thyroid cancer. Phase II study.
  Author(s): Bukowski RM, Brown L, Weick JK, Groppe CW, Purvis J.

Source: American Journal of Clinical Oncology : the Official Publication of the American Radium Society. 1983 October; 6(5): 579-81.
http://www.ncbi.nlm.nih.gov:80/entrez/query.fcgi?cmd=Retrieve&db=PubMed&list_uids=6193705&dopt=Abstract

- **Combined chemotherapy with bleomycin, adriamycin, and platinum in advanced thyroid cancer.**
  Author(s): De Besi P, Busnardo B, Toso S, Girelli ME, Nacamulli D, Simioni N, Casara D, Zorat P, Fiorentino MV.
  Source: J Endocrinol Invest. 1991 June; 14(6): 475-80.
  http://www.ncbi.nlm.nih.gov:80/entrez/query.fcgi?cmd=Retrieve&db=PubMed&list_uids=1723086&dopt=Abstract

- **Cytochrome c release is upstream to activation of caspase-9, caspase-8, and caspase-3 in the enhanced apoptosis of anaplastic thyroid cancer cells induced by manumycin and paclitaxel.**
  Author(s): Pan J, Xu G, Yeung SC.
  Source: The Journal of Clinical Endocrinology and Metabolism. 2001 October; 86(10): 4731-40.
  http://www.ncbi.nlm.nih.gov:80/entrez/query.fcgi?cmd=Retrieve&db=PubMed&list_uids=11600533&dopt=Abstract

- **Diagnostic fine-needle aspiration cytology and immunocytochemistry analysis of a primary thyroid lymphoma presenting as an anatomic emergency.**
  Author(s): Van D, Drijkoningen M, Oyen R, Vanfleteren E, Bouillon R.
  Source: Thyroid : Official Journal of the American Thyroid Association. 2002 February; 12(2): 169-73.
  http://www.ncbi.nlm.nih.gov:80/entrez/query.fcgi?cmd=Retrieve&db=PubMed&list_uids=11916287&dopt=Abstract

- **Differentiated thyroid cancer. Impact of adjuvant external radiotherapy in patients with perithyroidal tumor infiltration (stage pT4).**
  Author(s): Farahati J, Reiners C, Stuschke M, Muller SP, Stuben G, Sauerwein W, Sack H.
  Source: Cancer. 1996 January 1; 77(1): 172-80.
  http://www.ncbi.nlm.nih.gov:80/entrez/query.fcgi?cmd=Retrieve&db=PubMed&list_uids=8630926&dopt=Abstract

- **Effect of reserpine on salivary gland radioiodine uptake in thyroid cancer.**
  Author(s): Levy HA, Park CH.

Source: Clinical Nuclear Medicine. 1987 April; 12(4): 303-7.
http://www.ncbi.nlm.nih.gov:80/entrez/query.fcgi?cmd=Retrieve&db=PubMed&list_uids=3581610&dopt=Abstract

- **Effects of vinblastine and 5-fluorouracil on human glioma and thyroid cancer cell monolayers and spheroids.**
  Author(s): Nederman T.
  Source: Cancer Research. 1984 January; 44(1): 254-8.
  http://www.ncbi.nlm.nih.gov:80/entrez/query.fcgi?cmd=Retrieve&db=PubMed&list_uids=6690037&dopt=Abstract

- **Epidermal growth factor (EGF)- and transforming growth factor alpha-stimulated invasion and growth of follicular thyroid cancer cells can be blocked by antagonism to the EGF receptor and tyrosine kinase in vitro.**
  Author(s): Holting T, Siperstein AE, Clark OH, Duh QY.
  Source: European Journal of Endocrinology / European Federation of Endocrine Societies. 1995 February; 132(2): 229-35.
  http://www.ncbi.nlm.nih.gov:80/entrez/query.fcgi?cmd=Retrieve&db=PubMed&list_uids=7858744&dopt=Abstract

- **Evaluation of low-dose radioiodine ablation therapy in postsurgical thyroid cancer patients.**
  Author(s): Ramanna L, Waxman AD, Brachman MB, Tanasescu DE, Sensel N, Braunstein GD.
  Source: Clinical Nuclear Medicine. 1985 November; 10(11): 791-5.
  http://www.ncbi.nlm.nih.gov:80/entrez/query.fcgi?cmd=Retrieve&db=PubMed&list_uids=4075672&dopt=Abstract

- **Growth inhibitory effects of flavonoids in human thyroid cancer cell lines.**
  Author(s): Yin F, Giuliano AE, Van Herle AJ.
  Source: Thyroid : Official Journal of the American Thyroid Association. 1999 April; 9(4): 369-76.
  http://www.ncbi.nlm.nih.gov:80/entrez/query.fcgi?cmd=Retrieve&db=PubMed&list_uids=10319943&dopt=Abstract

- **Growth regulation of the human papillary thyroid cancer cell line by protein tyrosine kinase and cAMP-dependent protein kinase.**
  Author(s): Hishinuma A, Yamanaka T, Kasai K, So S, Bamba N, Shimoda SI.

Source: Endocr J. 1994 August; 41(4): 399-407.
http://www.ncbi.nlm.nih.gov:80/entrez/query.fcgi?cmd=Retrieve&db=PubMed&list_uids=8528355&dopt=Abstract

- **Influence of initial large dose on subsequent uptake of therapeutic radioiodine in thyroid cancer patients.**
  Author(s): Jeevanram RK, Shah DH, Sharma SM, Ganatra RD.
  Source: Int J Rad Appl Instrum B. 1986; 13(3): 277-9.
  http://www.ncbi.nlm.nih.gov:80/entrez/query.fcgi?cmd=Retrieve&db=PubMed&list_uids=3771260&dopt=Abstract

- **Initial experience with high-dose radioimmunotherapy of metastatic medullary thyroid cancer using 131I-MN-14 F(ab)2 anti-carcinoembryonic antigen MAb and AHSCR.**
  Author(s): Juweid ME, Hajjar G, Stein R, Sharkey RM, Herskovic T, Swayne LC, Suleiman S, Pereira M, Rubin AD, Goldenberg DM.
  Source: Journal of Nuclear Medicine : Official Publication, Society of Nuclear Medicine. 2000 January; 41(1): 93-103.
  http://www.ncbi.nlm.nih.gov:80/entrez/query.fcgi?cmd=Retrieve&db=PubMed&list_uids=10647610&dopt=Abstract

- **Iodine supplementation in Sweden and regional trends in thyroid cancer incidence by histopathologic type.**
  Author(s): Pettersson B, Coleman MP, Ron E, Adami HO.
  Source: International Journal of Cancer. Journal International Du Cancer. 1996 January 3; 65(1): 13-9.
  http://www.ncbi.nlm.nih.gov:80/entrez/query.fcgi?cmd=Retrieve&db=PubMed&list_uids=8543389&dopt=Abstract

- **Iodine-131 uptake in a patient with thyroid cancer and rheumatoid arthritis during acupuncture treatment.**
  Author(s): Otsuka N, Fukunaga M, Morita K, Ono S, Nagai K, Katagiri M, Harada T, Morita R.
  Source: Clinical Nuclear Medicine. 1990 January; 15(1): 29-31.
  http://www.ncbi.nlm.nih.gov:80/entrez/query.fcgi?cmd=Retrieve&db=PubMed&list_uids=2306894&dopt=Abstract

- **Large B-cell lymphoma of thyroid. Two cases with a marginal zone distribution of the neoplastic cells.**
  Author(s): Higgins JP, Warnke RA.

Source: Am J Clin Pathol. 2000 August; 114(2): 264-70.
http://www.ncbi.nlm.nih.gov:80/entrez/query.fcgi?cmd=Retrieve&db=PubMed&list_uids=10941342&dopt=Abstract

- **Low-dose and high-dose radioiodine in thyroid cancer.**
  Author(s): Ryo UY.
  Source: The American Journal of Medicine. 1977 July; 63(1): 167-8. No Abstract Available.
  http://www.ncbi.nlm.nih.gov:80/entrez/query.fcgi?cmd=Retrieve&db=PubMed&list_uids=879192&dopt=Abstract

- **Management of undifferentiated thyroid cancer.**
  Author(s): Ain KB.
  Source: Bailliere's Best Practice & Research. Clinical Endocrinology & Metabolism. 2000 December; 14(4): 615-29. Review.
  http://www.ncbi.nlm.nih.gov:80/entrez/query.fcgi?cmd=Retrieve&db=PubMed&list_uids=11289738&dopt=Abstract

- **Non-Hodgkin's lymphoma followed by plasmacytoma, both arising in A thyroid gland with Hashimoto's disease.**
  Author(s): Hasegawa Y, Itoh T, Tamagawa Y, Komeno T, Kojima H, Ninomiya H, Yatabe Y, Mori N, Nagasawa T.
  Source: Leukemia & Lymphoma. 1999 November; 35(5-6): 613-8.
  http://www.ncbi.nlm.nih.gov:80/entrez/query.fcgi?cmd=Retrieve&db=PubMed&list_uids=10609800&dopt=Abstract

- **Non-Hodgkin's lymphoma of the thyroid and adrenal glands.**
  Author(s): Lee DH, Park JH, Lee JJ, Chung IJ, Chung DJ, Chung MY, Lee TH.
  Source: Korean J Intern Med. 2000 January; 15(1): 76-80. Review.
  http://www.ncbi.nlm.nih.gov:80/entrez/query.fcgi?cmd=Retrieve&db=PubMed&list_uids=10714096&dopt=Abstract

- **Phase II study of etoposide (VP-16) in patients with thyroid cancer with no prior chemotherapy: an Eastern Cooperative Oncology Group Study (E1385).**
  Author(s): Leaf AN, Wolf BC, Kirkwood JM, Haselow RE.
  Source: Med Oncol. 2000 February; 17(1): 47-51.
  http://www.ncbi.nlm.nih.gov:80/entrez/query.fcgi?cmd=Retrieve&db=PubMed&list_uids=10713660&dopt=Abstract

- **Phytoestrogens and thyroid cancer risk: the San Francisco Bay Area thyroid cancer study.**
  Author(s): Horn-Ross PL, Hoggatt KJ, Lee MM.
  Source: Cancer Epidemiology, Biomarkers & Prevention : a Publication of the American Association for Cancer Research, Cosponsored by the American Society of Preventive Oncology. 2002 January; 11(1): 43-9.
  http://www.ncbi.nlm.nih.gov:80/entrez/query.fcgi?cmd=Retrieve&db=PubMed&list_uids=11815400&dopt=Abstract

- **Pregnancy following operative and complementary treatment of thyroid cancer.**
  Author(s): Pomorski L, Bartos M, Narebski J.
  Source: Zentralblatt Fur Gynakologie. 2000; 122(7): 383-6.
  http://www.ncbi.nlm.nih.gov:80/entrez/query.fcgi?cmd=Retrieve&db=PubMed&list_uids=10951709&dopt=Abstract

- **Primary thyroid lymphoma is a heterogeneous disease.**
  Author(s): Thieblemont C, Mayer A, Dumontet C, Barbier Y, Callet-Bauchu E, Felman P, Berger F, Ducottet X, Martin C, Salles G, Orgiazzi J, Coiffier B.
  Source: The Journal of Clinical Endocrinology and Metabolism. 2002 January; 87(1): 105-11.
  http://www.ncbi.nlm.nih.gov:80/entrez/query.fcgi?cmd=Retrieve&db=PubMed&list_uids=11788631&dopt=Abstract

- **Radioprotection of salivary glands by amifostine in high-dose radioiodine treatment. Results of a double-blinded, placebo-controlled study in patients with differentiated thyroid cancer.**
  Author(s): Bohuslavizki KH, Klutmann S, Brenner W, Kroger S, Buchert R, Bleckmann C, Mester J, Henze E, Clausen M.
  Source: Strahlentherapie Und Onkologie : Organ Der Deutschen Rontgengesellschaft . [et Al]. 1999 November; 175 Suppl 4: 6-12.
  http://www.ncbi.nlm.nih.gov:80/entrez/query.fcgi?cmd=Retrieve&db=PubMed&list_uids=10584133&dopt=Abstract

- **Resistance of [18f]-fluorodeoxyglucose-avid metastatic thyroid cancer lesions to treatment with high-dose radioactive iodine.**
  Author(s): Wang W, Larson SM, Tuttle RM, Kalaigian H, Kolbert K, Sonenberg M, Robbins RJ.

Source: Thyroid : Official Journal of the American Thyroid Association. 2001 December; 11(12): 1169-75.

http://www.ncbi.nlm.nih.gov:80/entrez/query.fcgi?cmd=Retrieve&db=PubMed&list_uids=12186505&dopt=Abstract

- **Resveratrol induces apoptosis in thyroid cancer cell lines via a MAPK- and p53-dependent mechanism.**
  Author(s): Shih A, Davis FB, Lin HY, Davis PJ.
  Source: The Journal of Clinical Endocrinology and Metabolism. 2002 March; 87(3): 1223-32.
  http://www.ncbi.nlm.nih.gov:80/entrez/query.fcgi?cmd=Retrieve&db=PubMed&list_uids=11889192&dopt=Abstract

- **Salivary gland protection by amifostine in high-dose radioiodine therapy of differentiated thyroid cancer.**
  Author(s): Bohuslavizki KH, Klutmann S, Bleckmann C, Brenner W, Lassmann S, Mester J, Henze E, Clausen M.
  Source: Strahlentherapie Und Onkologie : Organ Der Deutschen Rontgengesellschaft . [et Al]. 1999 February; 175(2): 57-61.
  http://www.ncbi.nlm.nih.gov:80/entrez/query.fcgi?cmd=Retrieve&db=PubMed&list_uids=10065139&dopt=Abstract

- **Selective cytotoxic activity of a novel ribonucleoside diphosphate reductase inhibitor MDL-101,731 against thyroid cancer in vitro.**
  Author(s): Kotchetkov R, Krivtchik AA, Cinatl J, Kornhuber B, Cinatl J Jr.
  Source: Folia Biol (Praha). 1999; 45(5): 185-91.
  http://www.ncbi.nlm.nih.gov:80/entrez/query.fcgi?cmd=Retrieve&db=PubMed&list_uids=10730887&dopt=Abstract

- **Spurious thyroid cancer metastasis: saliva contamination artifact in high dose iodine-131 metastases survey.**
  Author(s): Park HM, Tarver RD, Schauwecker DS, Burt R.
  Source: Journal of Nuclear Medicine : Official Publication, Society of Nuclear Medicine. 1986 May; 27(5): 634-6.
  http://www.ncbi.nlm.nih.gov:80/entrez/query.fcgi?cmd=Retrieve&db=PubMed&list_uids=3712080&dopt=Abstract

- **Surviving thyroid cancer. This silent cancer affects both young & old women.**
  Author(s): Biller L.

Source: Awhonn Lifelines / Association of Women's Health, Obstetric and Neonatal Nurses. 2002 June-July; 6(3): 280, 277-9. No Abstract Available.
http://www.ncbi.nlm.nih.gov:80/entrez/query.fcgi?cmd=Retrieve&db=PubMed&list_uids=12078573&dopt=Abstract

- **Swainsonine augments the cytotoxicity of human lymphokine-activated killer cells against autologous thyroid cancer cells.**
  Author(s): Fujieda S, Noda I, Saito H, Hoshino T, Yagita M.
  Source: Archives of Otolaryngology--Head & Neck Surgery. 1994 April; 120(4): 389-94.
  http://www.ncbi.nlm.nih.gov:80/entrez/query.fcgi?cmd=Retrieve&db=PubMed&list_uids=8166967&dopt=Abstract

- **Thyroid cancer.**
  Author(s): Rossi RL, Majlis S, Rossi RM.
  Source: The Surgical Clinics of North America. 2000 April; 80(2): 571-80. Review.
  http://www.ncbi.nlm.nih.gov:80/entrez/query.fcgi?cmd=Retrieve&db=PubMed&list_uids=10836007&dopt=Abstract

- **Thyrotropin stimulates invasion and growth of follicular thyroid cancer cells via PKC- rather than PKA-activation.**
  Author(s): Hoelting T, Tezelman S, Siperstein AE, Duh QY, Clark OH.
  Source: Biochemical and Biophysical Research Communications. 1993 September 30; 195(3): 1230-6.
  http://www.ncbi.nlm.nih.gov:80/entrez/query.fcgi?cmd=Retrieve&db=PubMed&list_uids=8216254&dopt=Abstract

- **Treating the patient with differentiated thyroid cancer with thyroglobulin-positive iodine-131 diagnostic scan-negative metastases: including comments on the role of serum thyroglobulin monitoring in tumor surveillance.**
  Author(s): Fatourechi V, Hay ID.
  Source: Semin Nucl Med. 2000 April; 30(2): 107-14. Review.
  http://www.ncbi.nlm.nih.gov:80/entrez/query.fcgi?cmd=Retrieve&db=PubMed&list_uids=10787191&dopt=Abstract

- **Treatment of anaplastic thyroid carcinoma with paclitaxel: phase 2 trial using ninety-six-hour infusion. Collaborative Anaplastic Thyroid Cancer Health Intervention Trials (CATCHIT) Group.**
  Author(s): Ain KB, Egorin MJ, DeSimone PA.

Source: Thyroid : Official Journal of the American Thyroid Association. 2000 July; 10(7): 587-94.
http://www.ncbi.nlm.nih.gov:80/entrez/query.fcgi?cmd=Retrieve&db=PubMed&list_uids=10958311&dopt=Abstract

Additional Web Resources

A number of additional Web sites offer encyclopedic information covering CAM and related topics. The following is a representative sample:

- Alternative Medicine Foundation, Inc.: **http://www.herbmed.org/**
- AOL: **http://search.aol.com/cat.adp?id=169&layer=&from=subcats**
- Chinese Medicine: **http://www.newcenturynutrition.com/**
- drkoop.com®: **http://www.drkoop.com/InteractiveMedicine/IndexC.html**
- Family Village: **http://www.familyvillage.wisc.edu/med_altn.htm**
- Google: **http://directory.google.com/Top/Health/Alternative/**
- Healthnotes: **http://www.thedacare.org/healthnotes/**
- Open Directory Project: **http://dmoz.org/Health/Alternative/**
- TPN.com: **http://www.tnp.com/**
- Yahoo.com: **http://dir.yahoo.com/Health/Alternative_Medicine/**
- WebMD®Health: **http://my.webmd.com/drugs_and_herbs**
- WellNet: **http://www.wellnet.ca/herbsa-c.htm**
- WholeHealthMD.com: **http://www.wholehealthmd.com/reflib/0,1529,,00.html**

The following is a specific Web list relating to thyroid cancer; please note that any particular subject below may indicate either a therapeutic use, or a contraindication (potential danger), and does not reflect an official recommendation:

- **General Overview**

    AIDS and HIV
    Source: Integrative Medicine Communications; www.onemedicine.com
    Hyperlink:
    http://www.drkoop.com/interactivemedicine/ConsConditions/HIVandAIDScc.html

    Amyloidosis
    Source: Integrative Medicine Communications; www.onemedicine.com
    Hyperlink:
    http://www.drkoop.com/interactivemedicine/ConsConditions/Amyloidosiscc.html

    Cancer Prevention and Diet
    Source: Healthnotes, Inc.; www.healthnotes.com
    Hyperlink:
    http://www.thedacare.org/healthnotes/Concern/Cancer_Diet.htm

    Celiac Disease
    Source: Healthnotes, Inc.; www.healthnotes.com
    Hyperlink:
    http://www.thedacare.org/healthnotes/Concern/Celiac_Disease.htm

    Cholesterol, High
    Source: Integrative Medicine Communications; www.onemedicine.com
    Hyperlink:
    http://www.drkoop.com/interactivemedicine/ConsConditions/Hypercholesterolemiacc.html

    Dermatitis Herpetiformis
    Source: Healthnotes, Inc.; www.healthnotes.com
    Hyperlink:
    http://www.thedacare.org/healthnotes/Concern/Dermatitis_Herpetiformis.htm

High Cholesterol
Source: Integrative Medicine Communications; www.onemedicine.com
Hyperlink: http://www.drkoop.com/interactivemedicine/ConsConditions/Hypercholesterolemiacc.html

HIV and AIDS
Source: Integrative Medicine Communications; www.onemedicine.com
Hyperlink: http://www.drkoop.com/interactivemedicine/ConsConditions/HIVandAIDScc.html

Hypercholesterolemia
Source: Integrative Medicine Communications; www.onemedicine.com
Hyperlink: http://www.drkoop.com/interactivemedicine/ConsConditions/Hypercholesterolemiacc.html

Lymphoma
Source: Integrative Medicine Communications; www.onemedicine.com
Hyperlink: http://www.drkoop.com/interactivemedicine/ConsConditions/Lymphomacc.html

Uveitis
Source: Integrative Medicine Communications; www.onemedicine.com
Hyperlink: http://www.drkoop.com/interactivemedicine/ConsConditions/Uveitiscc.html

- **Herbs and Supplements**

  ### Aloe
  Alternative names: Aloe vera L.
  Source: Alternative Medicine Foundation, Inc.; www.amfoundation.org
  Hyperlink: http://www.herbmed.org/

Aristolochia
Alternative names: Snakeroot, Guaco; Aristolochia sp
Source: Alternative Medicine Foundation, Inc.;
www.amfoundation.org
Hyperlink: http://www.herbmed.org/

Bryonia Bryony
Alternative names: Bryony; Bryonia sp.
Source: Alternative Medicine Foundation, Inc.;
www.amfoundation.org
Hyperlink: http://www.herbmed.org/

Coenzyme Q10
Source: Integrative Medicine Communications;
www.onemedicine.com
Hyperlink:
http://www.drkoop.com/interactivemedicine/ConsSupplements/CoenzymeQ10cs.html

CoQ10
Source: Integrative Medicine Communications;
www.onemedicine.com
Hyperlink:
http://www.drkoop.com/interactivemedicine/ConsSupplements/CoenzymeQ10cs.html

Curcuma
Alternative names: Turmeric; Curcuma longa L.
Source: Alternative Medicine Foundation, Inc.;
www.amfoundation.org
Hyperlink: http://www.herbmed.org/

Melatonin
Source: Integrative Medicine Communications;
www.onemedicine.com
Hyperlink:
http://www.drkoop.com/interactivemedicine/ConsSupplements/Melatonincs.html

Phytolacca
Alternative names: Poke root, Endod; Phytolacca dodecandra L.
Source: Alternative Medicine Foundation, Inc.;
www.amfoundation.org
Hyperlink: http://www.herbmed.org/

Thuja occid
Alternative names: Arbor Vitae; Thuja occidentalis
Source: Alternative Medicine Foundation, Inc.;
www.amfoundation.org
Hyperlink: http://www.herbmed.org/

Turmeric
Source: WholeHealthMD.com, LLC.; www.wholehealthmd.com
Hyperlink:
http://www.wholehealthmd.com/refshelf/substances_view/0,1525,
10062,00.html

Uncaria CatClaw
Alternative names: Cat's Claw, Uno de Gato; Uncaria tomentosa
(Willd.) D.C.
Source: Alternative Medicine Foundation, Inc.;
www.amfoundation.org
Hyperlink: http://www.herbmed.org/

Zingiber
Alternative names: Ginger; Zingiber officinale Roscoe
Source: Alternative Medicine Foundation, Inc.;
www.amfoundation.org
Hyperlink: http://www.herbmed.org/

General References

A good place to find general background information on CAM is the National Library of Medicine. It has prepared within the MEDLINEplus system an information topic page dedicated to complementary and alternative medicine. To access this page, go to the MEDLINEplus site at: **www.nlm.nih.gov/medlineplus/alternativemedicine.html.** This Web site provides a general overview of various topics and can lead to a number of general sources. The following additional references describe, in broad terms, alternative and complementary medicine (sorted alphabetically by title; hyperlinks provide rankings, information, and reviews at Amazon.com):

- **Alternative Medicine Definitive Guide to Cancer** by W. John Diamond, et al; Hardcover - 1120 pages Package edition (March 18, 1997), Alternativemedicine.Com Books; ISBN: 1887299017; http://www.amazon.com/exec/obidos/ASIN/1887299017/icongroupinterna

- **Beating Cancer With Nutrition - Revised** by Patrick Quillin, Noreen Quillin (Contributor); Paperback - 352 pages; Book & CD edition (January 1, 2001), Bookworld Services; ISBN: 0963837281; http://www.amazon.com/exec/obidos/ASIN/0963837281/icongroupinterna

- **Cancer: Increasing Your Odds for Survival - A Resource Guide for Integrating Mainstream, Alternative and Complementary Therapies** by David Bognar, Walter Cronkite; Paperback (August 1998), Hunter House; ISBN: 0897932471; http://www.amazon.com/exec/obidos/ASIN/0897932471/icongroupinterna

- **Choices in Healing** by Michael Lerner; Paperback - 696 pages; (February 28, 1996), MIT Press; ISBN: 0262621045; http://www.amazon.com/exec/obidos/ASIN/0262621045/icongroupinterna

- **The Gerson Therapy: The Amazing Nutritional Program for Cancer and Other Illnesses** by Charlotte Gerson, Morton Walker, D.P.M.; Paperback - 448 pages (October 2001), Kensington Publishing Corp.; ISBN: 1575666286; http://www.amazon.com/exec/obidos/ASIN/1575666286/icongroupinterna

- **Natural Compounds in Cancer Therapy** by John C. Boik; Paperback - 520 pages (March 2001), Oregon Medical Press; ISBN: 0964828014; http://www.amazon.com/exec/obidos/ASIN/0964828014/icongroupinterna

- **There's No Place Like Hope: A Guide to Beating Cancer in Mind-Sized Bites** by Vickie Girard, Dan Zadra (Editor); Hardcover - 161 pages (April 2001), Compendium Inc.; ISBN: 1888387416; http://www.amazon.com/exec/obidos/ASIN/1888387416/icongroupinterna

- **Your Life in Your Hands** by Jane A. Plant, Ph.D; Hardcover - 272 pages (December 13, 2000), St. Martins Press (Trade); ISBN: 0312275617; http://www.amazon.com/exec/obidos/ASIN/0312275617/icongroupinterna

For additional information on complementary and alternative medicine, ask your doctor or write to:

>National Institutes of Health
>National Center for Complementary and Alternative Medicine Clearinghouse
>P. O. Box 8218
>Silver Spring, MD 20907-8218

The following is a specific Web list relating to thyroid cancer; please note that any particular subject below may indicate either a therapeutic use, or a contraindication (potential danger), and does not reflect an official recommendation:

- **Vitamins**

    Folic Acid
    Source: Integrative Medicine Communications;
    www.onemedicine.com
    Hyperlink:
    http://www.drkoop.com/interactivemedicine/ConsSupplements/VitaminB9FolicAcidcs.html

    Vitamin B9 (Folic Acid)
    Alternative names: Folate, Folic Acid
    Source: Integrative Medicine Communications;
    www.onemedicine.com
    Hyperlink:
    http://www.drkoop.com/interactivemedicine/ConsSupplements/VitaminB9FolicAcidcs.html

- **Minerals**

    Folate
    Source: Integrative Medicine Communications;
    www.onemedicine.com
    Hyperlink:
    http://www.drkoop.com/interactivemedicine/ConsSupplements/VitaminB9FolicAcidcs.html

Iodine
Source: Healthnotes, Inc.; www.healthnotes.com
Hyperlink:
http://www.thedacare.org/healthnotes/Supp/Iodine.htm

Iodine
Source: Prima Communications, Inc.
Hyperlink: http://www.personalhealthzone.com/pg000153.html

Vanadium
Source: Healthnotes, Inc.; www.healthnotes.com
Hyperlink:
http://www.thedacare.org/healthnotes/Supp/Vanadium.htm

- **Food and Diet**

    ### High-Fiber Diet
    Source: Healthnotes, Inc.; www.healthnotes.com
    Hyperlink:
    http://www.thedacare.org/healthnotes/Diet/High_Fiber_Diet.htm

APPENDIX C. FINDING MEDICAL LIBRARIES

Overview

At a medical library you can find medical texts and reference books, consumer health publications, specialty newspapers and magazines, as well as medical journals. In this appendix, we show you how to quickly find a medical library in your area.

Preparation

Before going to the library, highlight the references mentioned in this sourcebook that you find interesting. Focus on those items that are not available via the Internet, and ask the reference librarian for help with your search. He or she may know of additional resources that could be helpful to you. Most importantly, your local public library and medical libraries have Interlibrary Loan programs with the National Library of Medicine (NLM), one of the largest medical collections in the world. According to the NLM, most of the literature in the general and historical collections of the National Library of Medicine is available on interlibrary loan to any library. NLM's interlibrary loan services are only available to libraries. If you would like to access NLM medical literature, then visit a library in your area that can request the publications for you.[118]

---

[118] Adapted from the NLM: **http://www.nlm.nih.gov/psd/cas/interlibrary.html**

226 Thyroid Cancer

Finding a Local Medical Library

The quickest method to locate medical libraries is to use the Internet-based directory published by the National Network of Libraries of Medicine (NN/LM). This network includes 4626 members and affiliates that provide many services to librarians, health professionals, and the public. To find a library in your area, simply visit **http://nnlm.gov/members/adv.html** or call 1-800-338-7657.

Medical Libraries Open to the Public

In addition to the NN/LM, the National Library of Medicine (NLM) lists a number of libraries that are generally open to the public and have reference facilities. The following is the NLM's list plus hyperlinks to each library Web site. These Web pages can provide information on hours of operation and other restrictions. The list below is a small sample of libraries recommended by the National Library of Medicine (sorted alphabetically by name of the U.S. state or Canadian province where the library is located):[119]

- **Alabama:** Health InfoNet of Jefferson County (Jefferson County Library Cooperative, Lister Hill Library of the Health Sciences), **http://www.uab.edu/infonet/**

- **Alabama:** Richard M. Scrushy Library (American Sports Medicine Institute), **http://www.asmi.org/LIBRARY.HTM**

- **Arizona:** Samaritan Regional Medical Center: The Learning Center (Samaritan Health System, Phoenix, Arizona), **http://www.samaritan.edu/library/bannerlibs.htm**

- **California:** Kris Kelly Health Information Center (St. Joseph Health System), **http://www.humboldt1.com/~kkhic/index.html**

- **California:** Community Health Library of Los Gatos (Community Health Library of Los Gatos), **http://www.healthlib.org/orgresources.html**

- **California:** Consumer Health Program and Services (CHIPS) (County of Los Angeles Public Library, Los Angeles County Harbor-UCLA Medical Center Library) - Carson, CA, **http://www.colapublib.org/services/chips.html**

- **California:** Gateway Health Library (Sutter Gould Medical Foundation)

- **California:** Health Library (Stanford University Medical Center), **http://www-med.stanford.edu/healthlibrary/**

---

[119] Abstracted from **http://www.nlm.nih.gov/medlineplus/libraries.html**.

- **California:** Patient Education Resource Center - Health Information and Resources (University of California, San Francisco), http://sfghdean.ucsf.edu/barnett/PERC/default.asp

- **California:** Redwood Health Library (Petaluma Health Care District), http://www.phcd.org/rdwdlib.html

- **California:** San José PlaneTree Health Library, http://planetreesanjose.org/

- **California:** Sutter Resource Library (Sutter Hospitals Foundation), http://go.sutterhealth.org/comm/resc-library/sac-resources.html

- **California:** University of California, Davis. Health Sciences Libraries

- **California:** ValleyCare Health Library & Ryan Comer Cancer Resource Center (ValleyCare Health System), http://www.valleycare.com/library.html

- **California:** Washington Community Health Resource Library (Washington Community Health Resource Library), http://www.healthlibrary.org/

- **Colorado:** William V. Gervasini Memorial Library (Exempla Healthcare), http://www.exempla.org/conslib.htm

- **Connecticut:** Hartford Hospital Health Science Libraries (Hartford Hospital), http://www.harthosp.org/library/

- **Connecticut:** Healthnet: Connecticut Consumer Health Information Center (University of Connecticut Health Center, Lyman Maynard Stowe Library), http://library.uchc.edu/departm/hnet/

- **Connecticut:** Waterbury Hospital Health Center Library (Waterbury Hospital), http://www.waterburyhospital.com/library/consumer.shtml

- **Delaware:** Consumer Health Library (Christiana Care Health System, Eugene du Pont Preventive Medicine & Rehabilitation Institute), http://www.christianacare.org/health_guide/health_guide_pmri_health_info.cfm

- **Delaware:** Lewis B. Flinn Library (Delaware Academy of Medicine), http://www.delamed.org/chls.html

- **Georgia:** Family Resource Library (Medical College of Georgia), http://cmc.mcg.edu/kids_families/fam_resources/fam_res_lib/frl.htm

- **Georgia:** Health Resource Center (Medical Center of Central Georgia), http://www.mccg.org/hrc/hrchome.asp

- **Hawaii:** Hawaii Medical Library: Consumer Health Information Service (Hawaii Medical Library), http://hml.org/CHIS/

- **Idaho:** DeArmond Consumer Health Library (Kootenai Medical Center), http://www.nicon.org/DeArmond/index.htm
- **Illinois:** Health Learning Center of Northwestern Memorial Hospital (Northwestern Memorial Hospital, Health Learning Center), http://www.nmh.org/health_info/hlc.html
- **Illinois:** Medical Library (OSF Saint Francis Medical Center), http://www.osfsaintfrancis.org/general/library/
- **Kentucky:** Medical Library - Services for Patients, Families, Students & the Public (Central Baptist Hospital), http://www.centralbap.com/education/community/library.htm
- **Kentucky:** University of Kentucky - Health Information Library (University of Kentucky, Chandler Medical Center, Health Information Library), http://www.mc.uky.edu/PatientEd/
- **Louisiana:** Alton Ochsner Medical Foundation Library (Alton Ochsner Medical Foundation), http://www.ochsner.org/library/
- **Louisiana:** Louisiana State University Health Sciences Center Medical Library-Shreveport, http://lib-sh.lsuhsc.edu/
- **Maine:** Franklin Memorial Hospital Medical Library (Franklin Memorial Hospital), http://www.fchn.org/fmh/lib.htm
- **Maine:** Gerrish-True Health Sciences Library (Central Maine Medical Center), http://www.cmmc.org/library/library.html
- **Maine:** Hadley Parrot Health Science Library (Eastern Maine Healthcare), http://www.emh.org/hll/hpl/guide.htm
- **Maine:** Maine Medical Center Library (Maine Medical Center), http://www.mmc.org/library/
- **Maine:** Parkview Hospital, http://www.parkviewhospital.org/communit.htm#Library
- **Maine:** Southern Maine Medical Center Health Sciences Library (Southern Maine Medical Center), http://www.smmc.org/services/service.php3?choice=10
- **Maine:** Stephens Memorial Hospital Health Information Library (Western Maine Health), http://www.wmhcc.com/hil_frame.html
- **Manitoba, Canada:** Consumer & Patient Health Information Service (University of Manitoba Libraries), http://www.umanitoba.ca/libraries/units/health/reference/chis.html
- **Manitoba, Canada:** J.W. Crane Memorial Library (Deer Lodge Centre), http://www.deerlodge.mb.ca/library/libraryservices.shtml

- **Maryland:** Health Information Center at the Wheaton Regional Library (Montgomery County, Md., Dept. of Public Libraries, Wheaton Regional Library), http://www.mont.lib.md.us/healthinfo/hic.asp

- **Massachusetts:** Baystate Medical Center Library (Baystate Health System), http://www.baystatehealth.com/1024/

- **Massachusetts:** Boston University Medical Center Alumni Medical Library (Boston University Medical Center), http://medlibwww.bu.edu/library/lib.html

- **Massachusetts:** Lowell General Hospital Health Sciences Library (Lowell General Hospital), http://www.lowellgeneral.org/library/HomePageLinks/WWW.htm

- **Massachusetts:** Paul E. Woodard Health Sciences Library (New England Baptist Hospital), http://www.nebh.org/health_lib.asp

- **Massachusetts:** St. Luke's Hospital Health Sciences Library (St. Luke's Hospital), http://www.southcoast.org/library/

- **Massachusetts:** Treadwell Library Consumer Health Reference Center (Massachusetts General Hospital), http://www.mgh.harvard.edu/library/chrcindex.html

- **Massachusetts:** UMass HealthNet (University of Massachusetts Medical School), http://healthnet.umassmed.edu/

- **Michigan:** Botsford General Hospital Library - Consumer Health (Botsford General Hospital, Library & Internet Services), http://www.botsfordlibrary.org/consumer.htm

- **Michigan:** Helen DeRoy Medical Library (Providence Hospital and Medical Centers), http://www.providence-hospital.org/library/

- **Michigan:** Marquette General Hospital - Consumer Health Library (Marquette General Hospital, Health Information Center), http://www.mgh.org/center.html

- **Michigan:** Patient Education Resouce Center - University of Michigan Cancer Center (University of Michigan Comprehensive Cancer Center), http://www.cancer.med.umich.edu/learn/leares.htm

- **Michigan:** Sladen Library & Center for Health Information Resources - Consumer Health Information, http://www.sladen.hfhs.org/library/consumer/index.html

- **Montana:** Center for Health Information (St. Patrick Hospital and Health Sciences Center), http://www.saintpatrick.org/chi/librarydetail.php3?ID=41

- **National:** Consumer Health Library Directory (Medical Library Association, Consumer and Patient Health Information Section), http://caphis.mlanet.org/directory/index.html

- **National:** National Network of Libraries of Medicine (National Library of Medicine) - provides library services for health professionals in the United States who do not have access to a medical library, http://nnlm.gov/

- **National:** NN/LM List of Libraries Serving the Public (National Network of Libraries of Medicine), http://nnlm.gov/members/

- **Nevada:** Health Science Library, West Charleston Library (Las Vegas Clark County Library District), http://www.lvccld.org/special_collections/medical/index.htm

- **New Hampshire:** Dartmouth Biomedical Libraries (Dartmouth College Library), http://www.dartmouth.edu/~biomed/resources.htmld/conshealth.htmld/

- **New Jersey:** Consumer Health Library (Rahway Hospital), http://www.rahwayhospital.com/library.htm

- **New Jersey:** Dr. Walter Phillips Health Sciences Library (Englewood Hospital and Medical Center), http://www.englewoodhospital.com/links/index.htm

- **New Jersey:** Meland Foundation (Englewood Hospital and Medical Center), http://www.geocities.com/ResearchTriangle/9360/

- **New York:** Choices in Health Information (New York Public Library) - NLM Consumer Pilot Project participant, http://www.nypl.org/branch/health/links.html

- **New York:** Health Information Center (Upstate Medical University, State University of New York), http://www.upstate.edu/library/hic/

- **New York:** Health Sciences Library (Long Island Jewish Medical Center), http://www.lij.edu/library/library.html

- **New York:** ViaHealth Medical Library (Rochester General Hospital), http://www.nyam.org/library/

- **Ohio:** Consumer Health Library (Akron General Medical Center, Medical & Consumer Health Library), http://www.akrongeneral.org/hwlibrary.htm

- **Oklahoma:** Saint Francis Health System Patient/Family Resource Center (Saint Francis Health System), http://www.sfh-tulsa.com/patientfamilycenter/default.asp

- **Oregon:** Planetree Health Resource Center (Mid-Columbia Medical Center), **http://www.mcmc.net/phrc/**
- **Pennsylvania:** Community Health Information Library (Milton S. Hershey Medical Center), **http://www.hmc.psu.edu/commhealth/**
- **Pennsylvania:** Community Health Resource Library (Geisinger Medical Center), **http://www.geisinger.edu/education/commlib.shtml**
- **Pennsylvania:** HealthInfo Library (Moses Taylor Hospital), **http://www.mth.org/healthwellness.html**
- **Pennsylvania:** Hopwood Library (University of Pittsburgh, Health Sciences Library System), **http://www.hsls.pitt.edu/chi/hhrcinfo.html**
- **Pennsylvania:** Koop Community Health Information Center (College of Physicians of Philadelphia), **http://www.collphyphil.org/kooppg1.shtml**
- **Pennsylvania:** Learning Resources Center - Medical Library (Susquehanna Health System), **http://www.shscares.org/services/lrc/index.asp**
- **Pennsylvania:** Medical Library (UPMC Health System), **http://www.upmc.edu/passavant/library.htm**
- **Quebec, Canada:** Medical Library (Montreal General Hospital), **http://ww2.mcgill.ca/mghlib/**
- **South Dakota:** Rapid City Regional Hospital - Health Information Center (Rapid City Regional Hospital, Health Information Center), **http://www.rcrh.org/education/LibraryResourcesConsumers.htm**
- **Texas:** Houston HealthWays (Houston Academy of Medicine-Texas Medical Center Library), **http://hhw.library.tmc.edu/**
- **Texas:** Matustik Family Resource Center (Cook Children's Health Care System), **http://www.cookchildrens.com/Matustik_Library.html**
- **Washington:** Community Health Library (Kittitas Valley Community Hospital), **http://www.kvch.com/**
- **Washington:** Southwest Washington Medical Center Library (Southwest Washington Medical Center), **http://www.swmedctr.com/Home/**

APPENDIX D. YOUR RIGHTS AND INSURANCE

Overview

Any patient with thyroid cancer faces a series of issues related more to the healthcare industry than to the medical condition itself. This appendix covers two important topics in this regard: your rights and responsibilities as a patient, and how to get the most out of your medical insurance plan.

Your Rights as a Patient

The President's Advisory Commission on Consumer Protection and Quality in the Healthcare Industry has created the following summary of your rights as a patient.[120]

Information Disclosure

Consumers have the right to receive accurate, easily understood information. Some consumers require assistance in making informed decisions about health plans, health professionals, and healthcare facilities. Such information includes:

- *Health plans.* Covered benefits, cost-sharing, and procedures for resolving complaints, licensure, certification, and accreditation status, comparable measures of quality and consumer satisfaction, provider network composition, the procedures that govern access to specialists and emergency services, and care management information.

---

[120] Adapted from Consumer Bill of Rights and Responsibilities: http://www.hcqualitycommission.gov/press/cbor.html#head1.

- *Health professionals.* Education, board certification, and recertification, years of practice, experience performing certain procedures, and comparable measures of quality and consumer satisfaction.

- *Healthcare facilities.* Experience in performing certain procedures and services, accreditation status, comparable measures of quality, worker, and consumer satisfaction, and procedures for resolving complaints.

- *Consumer assistance programs.* Programs must be carefully structured to promote consumer confidence and to work cooperatively with health plans, providers, payers, and regulators. Desirable characteristics of such programs are sponsorship that ensures accountability to the interests of consumers and stable, adequate funding.

Choice of Providers and Plans

Consumers have the right to a choice of healthcare providers that is sufficient to ensure access to appropriate high-quality healthcare. To ensure such choice, the Commission recommends the following:

- *Provider network adequacy.* All health plan networks should provide access to sufficient numbers and types of providers to assure that all covered services will be accessible without unreasonable delay -- including access to emergency services 24 hours a day and 7 days a week. If a health plan has an insufficient number or type of providers to provide a covered benefit with the appropriate degree of specialization, the plan should ensure that the consumer obtains the benefit outside the network at no greater cost than if the benefit were obtained from participating providers.

- *Women's health services.* Women should be able to choose a qualified provider offered by a plan -- such as gynecologists, certified nurse midwives, and other qualified healthcare providers -- for the provision of covered care necessary to provide routine and preventative women's healthcare services.

- *Access to specialists.* Consumers with complex or serious medical conditions who require frequent specialty care should have direct access to a qualified specialist of their choice within a plan's network of providers. Authorizations, when required, should be for an adequate number of direct access visits under an approved treatment plan.

- *Transitional care.* Consumers who are undergoing a course of treatment for a chronic or disabling condition (or who are in the second or third trimester of a pregnancy) at the time they involuntarily change health plans or at a time when a provider is terminated by a plan for other than cause should be able to continue seeing their current specialty providers for up to 90 days (or through completion of postpartum care) to allow for transition of care.

- *Choice of health plans.* Public and private group purchasers should, wherever feasible, offer consumers a choice of high-quality health insurance plans.

Access to Emergency Services

Consumers have the right to access emergency healthcare services when and where the need arises. Health plans should provide payment when a consumer presents to an emergency department with acute symptoms of sufficient severity--including severe pain--such that a "prudent layperson" could reasonably expect the absence of medical attention to result in placing that consumer's health in serious jeopardy, serious impairment to bodily functions, or serious dysfunction of any bodily organ or part.

Participation in Treatment Decisions

Consumers have the right and responsibility to fully participate in all decisions related to their healthcare. Consumers who are unable to fully participate in treatment decisions have the right to be represented by parents, guardians, family members, or other conservators. Physicians and other health professionals should:

- Provide patients with sufficient information and opportunity to decide among treatment options consistent with the informed consent process.

- Discuss all treatment options with a patient in a culturally competent manner, including the option of no treatment at all.

- Ensure that persons with disabilities have effective communications with members of the health system in making such decisions.

- Discuss all current treatments a consumer may be undergoing.

- Discuss all risks, benefits, and consequences to treatment or nontreatment.

- Give patients the opportunity to refuse treatment and to express preferences about future treatment decisions.

- Discuss the use of advance directives -- both living wills and durable powers of attorney for healthcare -- with patients and their designated family members.

- Abide by the decisions made by their patients and/or their designated representatives consistent with the informed consent process.

Health plans, health providers, and healthcare facilities should:

- Disclose to consumers factors -- such as methods of compensation, ownership of or interest in healthcare facilities, or matters of conscience -- that could influence advice or treatment decisions.

- Assure that provider contracts do not contain any so-called "gag clauses" or other contractual mechanisms that restrict healthcare providers' ability to communicate with and advise patients about medically necessary treatment options.

- Be prohibited from penalizing or seeking retribution against healthcare professionals or other health workers for advocating on behalf of their patients.

Respect and Nondiscrimination

Consumers have the right to considerate, respectful care from all members of the healthcare industry at all times and under all circumstances. An environment of mutual respect is essential to maintain a quality healthcare system. To assure that right, the Commission recommends the following:

- Consumers must not be discriminated against in the delivery of healthcare services consistent with the benefits covered in their policy, or as required by law, based on race, ethnicity, national origin, religion, sex, age, mental or physical disability, sexual orientation, genetic information, or source of payment.

- Consumers eligible for coverage under the terms and conditions of a health plan or program, or as required by law, must not be discriminated against in marketing and enrollment practices based on race, ethnicity, national origin, religion, sex, age, mental or physical disability, sexual orientation, genetic information, or source of payment.

Confidentiality of Health Information

Consumers have the right to communicate with healthcare providers in confidence and to have the confidentiality of their individually identifiable healthcare information protected. Consumers also have the right to review and copy their own medical records and request amendments to their records.

Complaints and Appeals

Consumers have the right to a fair and efficient process for resolving differences with their health plans, healthcare providers, and the institutions that serve them, including a rigorous system of internal review and an independent system of external review. A free copy of the Patient's Bill of Rights is available from the American Hospital Association.[121]

Patient Responsibilities

Treatment is a two-way street between you and your healthcare providers. To underscore the importance of finance in modern healthcare as well as your responsibility for the financial aspects of your care, the President's Advisory Commission on Consumer Protection and Quality in the Healthcare Industry has proposed that patients understand the following "Consumer Responsibilities."[122] In a healthcare system that protects consumers' rights, it is reasonable to expect and encourage consumers to assume certain responsibilities. Greater individual involvement by the consumer in his or her care increases the likelihood of achieving the best outcome and helps support a quality-oriented, cost-conscious environment. Such responsibilities include:

- Take responsibility for maximizing healthy habits such as exercising, not smoking, and eating a healthy diet.
- Work collaboratively with healthcare providers in developing and carrying out agreed-upon treatment plans.
- Disclose relevant information and clearly communicate wants and needs.
- Use your health insurance plan's internal complaint and appeal processes to address your concerns.
- Avoid knowingly spreading disease.

---

[121] To order your free copy of the Patient's Bill of Rights, telephone 312-422-3000 or visit the American Hospital Association's Web site: **http://www.aha.org**. Click on "Resource Center," go to "Search" at bottom of page, and then type in "Patient's Bill of Rights." The Patient's Bill of Rights is also available from Fax on Demand, at 312-422-2020, document number 471124.

[122] Adapted from **http://www.hcqualitycommission.gov/press/cbor.html#head1**.

- Recognize the reality of risks, the limits of the medical science, and the human fallibility of the healthcare professional.

- Be aware of a healthcare provider's obligation to be reasonably efficient and equitable in providing care to other patients and the community.

- Become knowledgeable about your health plan's coverage and options (when available) including all covered benefits, limitations, and exclusions, rules regarding use of network providers, coverage and referral rules, appropriate processes to secure additional information, and the process to appeal coverage decisions.

- Show respect for other patients and health workers.

- Make a good-faith effort to meet financial obligations.

- Abide by administrative and operational procedures of health plans, healthcare providers, and Government health benefit programs.

Choosing an Insurance Plan

There are a number of official government agencies that help consumers understand their healthcare insurance choices.[123] The U.S. Department of Labor, in particular, recommends ten ways to make your health benefits choices work best for you.[124]

1. Your options are important. There are many different types of health benefit plans. Find out which one your employer offers, then check out the plan, or plans, offered. Your employer's human resource office, the health plan administrator, or your union can provide information to help you match your needs and preferences with the available plans. The more information you have, the better your healthcare decisions will be.

2. Reviewing the benefits available. Do the plans offered cover preventive care, well-baby care, vision or dental care? Are there deductibles? Answers to these questions can help determine the out-of-pocket expenses you may face. Matching your needs and those of your family members will result in the best possible benefits. Cheapest may not always be best. Your goal is high quality health benefits.

---

[123] More information about quality across programs is provided at the following AHRQ Web site:
http://www.ahrq.gov/consumer/qntascii/qnthplan.htm .
[124] Adapted from the Department of Labor:
http://www.dol.gov/dol/pwba/public/pubs/health/top10-text.html.

3. Look for quality. The quality of healthcare services varies, but quality can be measured. You should consider the quality of healthcare in deciding among the healthcare plans or options available to you. Not all health plans, doctors, hospitals and other providers give the highest quality care. Fortunately, there is quality information you can use right now to help you compare your healthcare choices. Find out how you can measure quality. Consult the U.S. Department of Health and Human Services publication "Your Guide to Choosing Quality Health Care" on the Internet at **www.ahcpr.gov/consumer**.

4. Your plan's summary plan description (SPD) provides a wealth of information. Your health plan administrator can provide you with a copy of your plan's SPD. It outlines your benefits and your legal rights under the Employee Retirement Income Security Act (ERISA), the federal law that protects your health benefits. It should contain information about the coverage of dependents, what services will require a co-pay, and the circumstances under which your employer can change or terminate a health benefits plan. Save the SPD and all other health plan brochures and documents, along with memos or correspondence from your employer relating to health benefits.

5. Assess your benefit coverage as your family status changes. Marriage, divorce, childbirth or adoption, and the death of a spouse are all life events that may signal a need to change your health benefits. You, your spouse and dependent children may be eligible for a special enrollment period under provisions of the Health Insurance Portability and Accountability Act (HIPAA). Even without life-changing events, the information provided by your employer should tell you how you can change benefits or switch plans, if more than one plan is offered. If your spouse's employer also offers a health benefits package, consider coordinating both plans for maximum coverage.

6. Changing jobs and other life events can affect your health benefits. Under the Consolidated Omnibus Budget Reconciliation Act (COBRA), you, your covered spouse, and your dependent children may be eligible to purchase extended health coverage under your employer's plan if you lose your job, change employers, get divorced, or upon occurrence of certain other events. Coverage can range from 18 to 36 months depending on your situation. COBRA applies to most employers with 20 or more workers and requires your plan to notify you of your rights. Most plans require eligible individuals to make their COBRA election within 60 days of the plan's notice. Be sure to follow up with your plan sponsor if you don't receive notice, and make sure you respond within the allotted time.

7. HIPAA can also help if you are changing jobs, particularly if you have a medical condition. HIPAA generally limits pre-existing condition exclusions to a maximum of 12 months (18 months for late enrollees). HIPAA also requires this maximum period to be reduced by the length of time you had prior "creditable coverage." You should receive a certificate documenting your prior creditable coverage from your old plan when coverage ends.

8. Plan for retirement. Before you retire, find out what health benefits, if any, extend to you and your spouse during your retirement years. Consult with your employer's human resources office, your union, the plan administrator, and check your SPD. Make sure there is no conflicting information among these sources about the benefits you will receive or the circumstances under which they can change or be eliminated. With this information in hand, you can make other important choices, like finding out if you are eligible for Medicare and Medigap insurance coverage.

9. Know how to file an appeal if your health benefits claim is denied. Understand how your plan handles grievances and where to make appeals of the plan's decisions. Keep records and copies of correspondence. Check your health benefits package and your SPD to determine who is responsible for handling problems with benefit claims. Contact PWBA for customer service assistance if you are unable to obtain a response to your complaint.

10. You can take steps to improve the quality of the healthcare and the health benefits you receive. Look for and use things like Quality Reports and Accreditation Reports whenever you can. Quality reports may contain consumer ratings -- how satisfied consumers are with the doctors in their plan, for instance-- and clinical performance measures -- how well a healthcare organization prevents and treats illness. Accreditation reports provide information on how accredited organizations meet national standards, and often include clinical performance measures. Look for these quality measures whenever possible. Consult "Your Guide to Choosing Quality Health Care" on the Internet at **www.ahcpr.gov/consumer**.

Medicare and Medicaid

Illness strikes both rich and poor families. For low-income families, Medicaid is available to defer the costs of treatment. The Health Care Financing Administration (HCFA) administers Medicare, the nation's largest health insurance program, which covers 39 million Americans. In the following pages, you will learn the basics about Medicare insurance as well as useful contact information on how to find more in-depth information about Medicaid.[125]

Who is Eligible for Medicare?

Generally, you are eligible for Medicare if you or your spouse worked for at least 10 years in Medicare-covered employment and you are 65 years old and a citizen or permanent resident of the United States. You might also qualify for coverage if you are under age 65 but have a disability or End-Stage Renal disease (permanent kidney failure requiring dialysis or transplant). Here are some simple guidelines:

You can get Part A at age 65 without having to pay premiums if:

- You are already receiving retirement benefits from Social Security or the Railroad Retirement Board.
- You are eligible to receive Social Security or Railroad benefits but have not yet filed for them.
- You or your spouse had Medicare-covered government employment.

If you are under 65, you can get Part A without having to pay premiums if:

- You have received Social Security or Railroad Retirement Board disability benefit for 24 months.
- You are a kidney dialysis or kidney transplant patient.

Medicare has two parts:
- Part A (Hospital Insurance). Most people do not have to pay for Part A.
- Part B (Medical Insurance). Most people pay monthly for Part B.

Part A (Hospital Insurance)

Helps Pay For: Inpatient hospital care, care in critical access hospitals (small facilities that give limited outpatient and inpatient services to people in rural areas) and skilled nursing facilities, hospice care, and some home healthcare.

---

[125] This section has been adapted from the Official U.S. Site for Medicare Information: http://www.medicare.gov/Basics/Overview.asp.

Cost: Most people get Part A automatically when they turn age 65. You do not have to pay a monthly payment called a premium for Part A because you or a spouse paid Medicare taxes while you were working.

If you (or your spouse) did not pay Medicare taxes while you were working and you are age 65 or older, you still may be able to buy Part A. If you are not sure you have Part A, look on your red, white, and blue Medicare card. It will show "Hospital Part A" on the lower left corner of the card. You can also call the Social Security Administration toll free at 1-800-772-1213 or call your local Social Security office for more information about buying Part A. If you get benefits from the Railroad Retirement Board, call your local RRB office or 1-800-808-0772. For more information, call your Fiscal Intermediary about Part A bills and services. The phone number for the Fiscal Intermediary office in your area can be obtained from the following Web site: **http://www.medicare.gov/Contacts/home.asp**.

Part B (Medical Insurance)

Helps Pay For: Doctors, services, outpatient hospital care, and some other medical services that Part A does not cover, such as the services of physical and occupational therapists, and some home healthcare. Part B helps pay for covered services and supplies when they are medically necessary.

Cost: As of 2001, you pay the Medicare Part B premium of $50.00 per month. In some cases this amount may be higher if you did not choose Part B when you first became eligible at age 65. The cost of Part B may go up 10% for each 12-month period that you were eligible for Part B but declined coverage, except in special cases. You will have to pay the extra 10% cost for the rest of your life.

Enrolling in Part B is your choice. You can sign up for Part B anytime during a 7-month period that begins 3 months before you turn 65. Visit your local Social Security office, or call the Social Security Administration at 1-800-772-1213 to sign up. If you choose to enroll in Part B, the premium is usually taken out of your monthly Social Security, Railroad Retirement, or Civil Service Retirement payment. If you do not receive any of the above payments, Medicare sends you a bill for your part B premium every 3 months. You should receive your Medicare premium bill in the mail by the 10th of the month. If you do not, call the Social Security Administration at 1-800-772-1213, or your local Social Security office. If you get benefits from the Railroad Retirement Board, call your local RRB office or 1-800-808-0772. For more information, call your Medicare carrier about bills and services. The phone number for the Medicare carrier in your area can be found at the following Web site: **http://www.medicare.gov/Contacts/home.asp**. You may have choices in how you get your healthcare including the Original Medicare Plan, Medicare Managed Care Plans (like HMOs), and Medicare Private Fee-for-Service Plans.

Medicaid

Medicaid is a joint federal and state program that helps pay medical costs for some people with low incomes and limited resources. Medicaid programs vary from state to state. People on Medicaid may also get coverage for nursing home care and outpatient prescription drugs which are not covered by Medicare. You can find more information about Medicaid on the HCFA.gov Web site at **http://www.hcfa.gov/medicaid/medicaid.htm**.

States also have programs that pay some or all of Medicare's premiums and may also pay Medicare deductibles and coinsurance for certain people who have Medicare and a low income. To qualify, you must have:

- Part A (Hospital Insurance),
- Assets, such as bank accounts, stocks, and bonds that are not more than $4,000 for a single person, or $6,000 for a couple, and
- A monthly income that is below certain limits.

For more information on these programs, look at the Medicare Savings Programs brochure, **http://www.medicare.gov/Library/PDFNavigation/PDFInterim.asp?Language=English&Type=Pub&PubID=10126**. There are also Prescription Drug Assistance Programs available. Find information on these programs which offer discounts or free medications to individuals in need at **http://www.medicare.gov/Prescription/Home.asp**.

Financial Assistance for Cancer Care[126]

Cancer imposes heavy economic burdens on both patients and their families. For many people, a portion of medical expenses is paid by their health insurance plan. For individuals who do not have health insurance or who need financial assistance to cover health care costs, resources are available,

---

[126] Adapted from the NCI: **http://cis.nci.nih.gov/fact/8_3.htm**.

including government-sponsored programs and services supported by voluntary organizations.

Cancer patients and their families should discuss any concerns they may have about health care costs with their physician, medical social worker, or the business office of their hospital or clinic.

The organizations and resources listed below may offer financial assistance. Organizations that provide publications in Spanish or have Spanish-speaking staff have been identified.

- The American Cancer Society (ACS) office can provide the telephone number of the local ACS office serving your area. The local ACS office may offer reimbursement for expenses related to cancer treatment including transportation, medicine, and medical supplies. The ACS also offers programs that help cancer patients, family members, and friends cope with the emotional challenges they face. Some publications are available in Spanish. Spanish-speaking staff are available. Telephone: 1-800-ACS-2345 (1-800-227-2345). Web site: **http://www.cancer.org**

- The *AVONCares* Program for Medically Underserved Women provides financial assistance and relevant education and support to low income, under- and uninsured, underserved women throughout the country in need of diagnostic and/or related services (transportation, child care, and social support) for the treatment of breast, cervical, and ovarian cancers. Telephone: 1-800-813-HOPE (1-800-813-4673). Web site: **http://www.cancercare.org**.

Community voluntary agencies and service organizations such as the Salvation Army, Lutheran Social Services, Jewish Social Services, Catholic Charities, and the Lions Club may offer help. These organizations are listed in your local phone directory. Some churches and synagogues may provide financial help or services to their members.
Fundraising is another mechanism to consider. Some patients find that friends, family, and community members are willing to contribute financially if they are aware of a difficult situation. Contact your local library for information about how to organize fundraising efforts.

General assistance programs provide food, housing, prescription drugs, and other medical expenses for those who are not eligible for other programs. Funds are often limited. Information can be obtained by contacting your state or local Department of Social Services; this number is found in the local telephone directory.

Hill-Burton is a program through which hospitals receive construction funds from the Federal Government. Hospitals that receive Hill-Burton funds are required by law to provide some services to people who cannot afford to pay for their hospitalization. Information about which facilities are part of this program is available by calling the toll-free number or visiting the Web site shown below. A brochure about the program is available in Spanish. Telephone: 1-800-638-0742. Web site: **http://www.hrsa.gov/osp/dfcr/obtain/consfaq.htm**.

Income Tax Deductions

Medical costs that are not covered by insurance policies sometimes can be deducted from annual income before taxes. Examples of tax deductible expenses might include mileage for trips to and from medical appointments, out-of-pocket costs for treatment, prescription drugs or equipment, and the cost of meals during lengthy medical visits. The local Internal Revenue Service office, tax consultants, or certified public accountants can determine medical costs that are tax deductible. These telephone numbers are available in the local telephone directory. Web site: **http://www.irs.ustreas.gov**.

The Patient Advocate Foundation

The Patient Advocate Foundation (PAF) is a national nonprofit organization that provides education, legal counseling, and referrals to cancer patients and survivors concerning managed care, insurance, financial issues, job discrimination, and debt crisis matters. Telephone: 1-800-532-5274. **Web site: http://www.patientadvocate.org**.

Patient Assistance Programs are offered by some pharmaceutical manufacturers to help pay for medications. To learn whether a specific drug might be available at reduced cost through such a program, talk with a physician or a medical social worker.

Transportation

There are nonprofit organizations that arrange free or reduced cost air transportation for cancer patients going to or from cancer treatment centers. Financial need is not always a requirement. To find out about these programs, talk with a medical social worker. Ground transportation services may be offered or mileage reimbursed through the local ACS or your state or local Department of Social Services.

Veterans Benefits

Eligible veterans and their dependents may receive cancer treatment at a Veterans Administration Medical Center. Treatment for service-connected conditions is provided, and treatment for other conditions may be available based on the veteran's financial need. Some publications are available in Spanish. Spanish-speaking staff are available in some offices. Telephone: 1-877-222-VETS. Web site: **http://www.va.gov/vbs/health**.

NORD's Medication Assistance Programs

Finally, the National Organization for Rare Disorders, Inc. (NORD) administers medication programs sponsored by humanitarian-minded pharmaceutical and biotechnology companies to help uninsured or under-insured individuals secure life-saving or life-sustaining drugs.[127] NORD programs ensure that certain vital drugs are available "to those individuals whose income is too high to qualify for Medicaid but too low to pay for their prescribed medications." The program has standards for fairness, equity, and unbiased eligibility. It currently covers some 14 programs for nine pharmaceutical companies. NORD also offers early access programs for investigational new drugs (IND) under the approved "Treatment INDs" programs of the Food and Drug Administration (FDA). In these programs, a limited number of individuals can receive investigational drugs that have yet to be approved by the FDA. These programs are generally designed for rare diseases or disorders. For more information, visit **www.rarediseases.org**.

---

[127] Adapted from NORD: **http://www.rarediseases.org/cgi-bin/nord/progserv#patient?id=rPIzL9oD&mv_pc=30**.

Additional Resources

In addition to the references already listed in this chapter, you may need more information on health insurance, hospitals, or the healthcare system in general. The NIH has set up an excellent guidance Web site that addresses these and other issues. Topics include:[128]

- Health Insurance:
  http://www.nlm.nih.gov/medlineplus/healthinsurance.html
- Health Statistics:
  http://www.nlm.nih.gov/medlineplus/healthstatistics.html
- HMO and Managed Care:
  http://www.nlm.nih.gov/medlineplus/managedcare.html
- Hospice Care: **http://www.nlm.nih.gov/medlineplus/hospicecare.html**
- Medicaid: **http://www.nlm.nih.gov/medlineplus/medicaid.html**
- Medicare: **http://www.nlm.nih.gov/medlineplus/medicare.html**
- Nursing Homes and Long-term Care:
  http://www.nlm.nih.gov/medlineplus/nursinghomes.html
- Patient's Rights, Confidentiality, Informed Consent, Ombudsman Programs, Privacy and Patient Issues:
  http://www.nlm.nih.gov/medlineplus/patientissues.html
- Veteran's Health, Persian Gulf War, Gulf War Syndrome, Agent Orange:
  http://www.nlm.nih.gov/medlineplus/veteranshealth.html

Vocabulary Builder

Amifostine: A drug used as a chemoprotective drug to control some of the side effects of chemotherapy and radiation therapy. [NIH]

Antigen: Any substance which is capable, under appropriate conditions, of inducing a specific immune response and of reacting with the products of that response, that is, with specific antibody or specifically sensitized T-lymphocytes, or both. Antigens may be soluble substances, such as toxins and foreign proteins, or particulate, such as bacteria and tissue cells; however, only the portion of the protein or polysaccharide molecule known as the antigenic determinant (q.v.) combines with antibody or a specific

---

[128] You can access this information at:
http://www.nlm.nih.gov/medlineplus/healthsystem.html.

receptor on a lymphocyte. Abbreviated Ag. [EU]

Biomarkers: Substances sometimes found in an increased amount in the blood, other body fluids, or tissues and that may suggest the presence of some types of cancer. Biomarkers include CA 125 (ovarian cancer), CA 15-3 (breast cancer), CEA (ovarian, lung, breast, pancreas, and GI tract cancers), and PSA (prostate cancer). Also called tumor markers. [NIH]

Coenzyme: An organic nonprotein molecule, frequently a phosphorylated derivative of a water-soluble vitamin, that binds with the protein molecule (apoenzyme) to form the active enzyme (holoenzyme). [EU]

Contamination: The soiling or pollution by inferior material, as by the introduction of organisms into a wound, or sewage into a stream. [EU]

Dermatitis: Inflammation of the skin. [NIH]

Fluorouracil: An anticancer drug that belongs to the family of drugs called antimetabolites. [NIH]

Glioma: A cancer of the brain that comes from glial, or supportive, cells. [NIH]

Infiltration: The diffusion or accumulation in a tissue or cells of substances not normal to it or in amounts of the normal. Also, the material so accumulated. [EU]

Inoperable: Not suitable to be operated upon. [EU]

Plasmacytoma: Cancer of the plasma cells (white blood cells that produce antibodies) that may turn into multiple myeloma. [NIH]

Psychotherapy: A generic term for the treatment of mental illness or emotional disturbances primarily by verbal or nonverbal communication. [NIH]

Radioimmunotherapy: Treatment with a radioactive substance that is linked to an antibody that will attach to the tumor when injected into the body. [NIH]

Radiology: The use of radiation (such as x-rays) or other imaging technologies (such as ultrasound and magnetic resonance imaging) to diagnose or treat disease. [NIH]

Radium: Radium. A radioactive element of the alkaline earth series of metals. It has the atomic symbol Ra, atomic number 88, and atomic weight 226. Radium is the product of the disintegration of uranium and is present in pitchblende and all ores containing uranium. It is used clinically as a source of beta and gamma-rays in radiotherapy, particularly brachytherapy. [NIH]

Reserpine: An alkaloid found in the roots of Rauwolfia serpentina and R. vomitoria. Reserpine inhibits the uptake of norepinephrine into storage vesicles resulting in depletion of catecholamines and serotonin from central and peripheral axon terminals. It has been used as an antihypertensive and an antipsychotic as well as a research tool, but its adverse effects limit its clinical use. [NIH]

Uveitis: An inflammation of part or all of the uvea, the middle (vascular) tunic of the eye, and commonly involving the other tunics (the sclera and cornea, and the retina). [EU]

Vanadium: Vanadium. A metallic element with the atomic symbol V, atomic number 23, and atomic weight 50.94. It is used in the manufacture of vanadium steel. Prolonged exposure can lead to chronic intoxication caused by absorption usually via the lungs. [NIH]

ONLINE GLOSSARIES

The Internet provides access to a number of free-to-use medical dictionaries and glossaries. The National Library of Medicine has compiled the following list of online dictionaries:

- ADAM Medical Encyclopedia (A.D.A.M., Inc.), comprehensive medical reference: **http://www.nlm.nih.gov/medlineplus/encyclopedia.html**

- MedicineNet.com Medical Dictionary (MedicineNet, Inc.): **http://www.medterms.com/Script/Main/hp.asp**

- Merriam-Webster Medical Dictionary (Inteli-Health, Inc.): **http://www.intelihealth.com/IH/**

- Multilingual Glossary of Technical and Popular Medical Terms in Eight European Languages (European Commission) - Danish, Dutch, English, French, German, Italian, Portuguese, and Spanish: **http://allserv.rug.ac.be/~rvdstich/eugloss/welcome.html**

- On-line Medical Dictionary (CancerWEB): **http://www.graylab.ac.uk/omd/**

- Technology Glossary (National Library of Medicine) - Health Care Technology: **http://www.nlm.nih.gov/nichsr/ta101/ta10108.htm**

- Terms and Definitions (Office of Rare Diseases): **http://rarediseases.info.nih.gov/ord/glossary_a-e.html**

Beyond these, MEDLINEplus contains a very user-friendly encyclopedia covering every aspect of medicine (licensed from A.D.A.M., Inc.). The ADAM Medical Encyclopedia Web site address is **http://www.nlm.nih.gov/medlineplus/encyclopedia.html**. ADAM is also available on commercial Web sites such as drkoop.com (**http://www.drkoop.com/**) and Web MD (**http://my.webmd.com/adam/asset/adam_disease_articles/a_to_z/a**). Topics of interest can be researched by using keywords before continuing elsewhere, as these basic definitions and concepts will be useful in more advanced areas of research. You may choose to print various pages specifically relating to thyroid cancer and keep them on file. The NIH, in particular, suggests that patients with thyroid cancer visit the following Web sites in the ADAM Medical Encyclopedia:

- **Basic Guidelines for Thyroid Cancer**

    Thyroid cancer
    Web site:
    http://www.nlm.nih.gov/medlineplus/ency/article/001213.htm

- **Signs & Symptoms for Thyroid Cancer**

    Breathing difficulties
    Web site:
    http://www.nlm.nih.gov/medlineplus/ency/article/003075.htm

    Constipation
    Web site:
    http://www.nlm.nih.gov/medlineplus/ency/article/003125.htm

    Cough
    Web site:
    http://www.nlm.nih.gov/medlineplus/ency/article/003072.htm

    Diarrhea
    Web site:
    http://www.nlm.nih.gov/medlineplus/ency/article/003126.htm

    Hoarseness or changing voice
    Web site:
    http://www.nlm.nih.gov/medlineplus/ency/article/003054.htm

    Neck swelling
    Web site:
    http://www.nlm.nih.gov/medlineplus/ency/article/003262.htm

    Nodules
    Web site:
    http://www.nlm.nih.gov/medlineplus/ency/article/003230.htm

    Stress
    Web site:
    http://www.nlm.nih.gov/medlineplus/ency/article/003211.htm

Swelling
Web site:
http://www.nlm.nih.gov/medlineplus/ency/article/003103.htm

- **Diagnostics and Tests for Thyroid Cancer**

ALT
Web site:
http://www.nlm.nih.gov/medlineplus/ency/article/003473.htm

ANA
Web site:
http://www.nlm.nih.gov/medlineplus/ency/article/003535.htm

Biopsy
Web site:
http://www.nlm.nih.gov/medlineplus/ency/article/003416.htm

Calcitonin
Web site:
http://www.nlm.nih.gov/medlineplus/ency/article/003699.htm

CEA
Web site:
http://www.nlm.nih.gov/medlineplus/ency/article/003574.htm

Dexamethasone suppression test
Web site:
http://www.nlm.nih.gov/medlineplus/ency/article/003694.htm

Laryngoscopy
Web site:
http://www.nlm.nih.gov/medlineplus/ency/article/003851.htm

Serum calcitonin
Web site:
http://www.nlm.nih.gov/medlineplus/ency/article/003699.htm

T3
Web site:
http://www.nlm.nih.gov/medlineplus/ency/article/003687.htm

T4
Web site:
http://www.nlm.nih.gov/medlineplus/ency/article/003517.htm

Thyroid biopsy
Web site:
http://www.nlm.nih.gov/medlineplus/ency/article/003901.htm

Thyroid scan
Web site:
http://www.nlm.nih.gov/medlineplus/ency/article/003829.htm

Ultrasound
Web site:
http://www.nlm.nih.gov/medlineplus/ency/article/003336.htm

Ultrasound of the thyroid
Web site:
http://www.nlm.nih.gov/medlineplus/ency/article/003776.htm

- **Background Topics for Thyroid Cancer**

    Bleeding
    Web site:
    http://www.nlm.nih.gov/medlineplus/ency/article/000045.htm

    Cancer - support group
    Web site:
    http://www.nlm.nih.gov/medlineplus/ency/article/002166.htm

    Chemotherapy
    Web site:
    http://www.nlm.nih.gov/medlineplus/ency/article/002324.htm

    Chronic
    Web site:
    http://www.nlm.nih.gov/medlineplus/ency/article/002312.htm

    Incidence
    Web site:
    http://www.nlm.nih.gov/medlineplus/ency/article/002387.htm

Laryngoscopy
Web site:
http://www.nlm.nih.gov/medlineplus/ency/article/003851.htm

Malignancy
Web site:
http://www.nlm.nih.gov/medlineplus/ency/article/002253.htm

Metastasis
Web site:
http://www.nlm.nih.gov/medlineplus/ency/article/002260.htm

Physical examination
Web site:
http://www.nlm.nih.gov/medlineplus/ency/article/002274.htm

Radiation therapy
Web site:
http://www.nlm.nih.gov/medlineplus/ency/article/001918.htm

Support group
Web site:
http://www.nlm.nih.gov/medlineplus/ency/article/002150.htm

Online Dictionary Directories

The following are additional online directories compiled by the National Library of Medicine, including a number of specialized medical dictionaries and glossaries:

- Medical Dictionaries: Medical & Biological (World Health Organization):
  http://www.who.int/hlt/virtuallibrary/English/diction.htm#Medical

- MEL-Michigan Electronic Library List of Online Health and Medical Dictionaries (Michigan Electronic Library):
  http://mel.lib.mi.us/health/health-dictionaries.html

- Patient Education: Glossaries (DMOZ Open Directory Project):
  http://dmoz.org/Health/Education/Patient_Education/Glossaries/

- Web of Online Dictionaries (Bucknell University):
  http://www.yourdictionary.com/diction5.html#medicine

THYROID CANCER GLOSSARY

The following is a complete glossary of terms used in this sourcebook. The definitions are derived from official public sources including the National Institutes of Health [NIH] and the European Union [EU]. After this glossary, we list a number of additional hardbound and electronic glossaries and dictionaries that you may wish to consult.

Abdomen: The part of the body that contains the pancreas, stomach, intestines, liver, gallbladder, and other organs. [NIH]

Acne: A disorder of the skin marked by inflammation of oil glands and hair glands. [NIH]

Adenocarcinoma: Cancer that begins in cells that line certain internal organs and that have glandular (secretory) properties. [NIH]

Adenoma: A noncancerous tumor. [NIH]

Adenosine: A nucleoside that is composed of adenine and d-ribose. Adenosine or adenosine derivatives play many important biological roles in addition to being components of DNA and RNA. Adenosine itself is a neurotransmitter. [NIH]

Adenovirus: A group of viruses that cause respiratory tract and eye infections. Adenoviruses used in gene therapy are altered to carry a specific tumor-fighting gene. [NIH]

Agonists: Drugs that trigger an action from a cell or another drug. [NIH]

Allogeneic: Taken from different individuals of the same species. [NIH]

Amifostine: A drug used as a chemoprotective drug to control some of the side effects of chemotherapy and radiation therapy. [NIH]

Amyloidosis: A group of diseases in which protein is deposited in specific organs (localized amyloidosis) or throughout the body (systemic amyloidosis). Amyloidosis may be either primary (with no known cause) or secondary (caused by another disease, including some types of cancer). Generally, primary amyloidosis affects the nerves, skin, tongue, joints, heart, and liver; secondary amyloidosis often affects the spleen, kidneys, liver, and adrenal glands. [NIH]

Analog: In chemistry, a substance that is similar, but not identical, to another. [NIH]

Anaplastic: A term used to describe cancer cells that divide rapidly and bear little or no resemblance to normal cells. [NIH]

Androgenic: Producing masculine characteristics. [EU]

Angiogenesis: Blood vessel formation. Tumor angiogenesis is the growth of blood vessels from surrounding tissue to a solid tumor. This is caused by the release of chemicals by the tumor. [NIH]

Antibody: A type of protein made by certain white blood cells in response to a foreign substance (antigen). Each antibody can bind to only a specific antigen. The purpose of this binding is to help destroy the antigen. Antibodies can work in several ways, depending on the nature of the antigen. Some antibodies destroy antigens directly. Others make it easier for white blood cells to destroy the antigen. [NIH]

Antigen: Any substance which is capable, under appropriate conditions, of inducing a specific immune response and of reacting with the products of that response, that is, with specific antibody or specifically sensitized T-lymphocytes, or both. Antigens may be soluble substances, such as toxins and foreign proteins, or particulate, such as bacteria and tissue cells; however, only the portion of the protein or polysaccharide molecule known as the antigenic determinant (q.v.) combines with antibody or a specific receptor on a lymphocyte. Abbreviated Ag. [EU]

Antineoplastons: Substances isolated from normal human blood and urine being tested as a type of treatment for some tumors and AIDS. [NIH]

Aplidine: An anticancer drug obtained from a marine animal. [NIH]

Apoptosis: A normal series of events in a cell that leads to its death. [NIH]

Aqueous: Having to do with water. [NIH]

Aspirate: Fluid withdrawn from a lump, often a cyst, or a nipple. [NIH]

Aspiration: Removal of fluid from a lump, often a cyst, with a needle and a syringe. [NIH]

Aspirin: A drug that reduces pain, fever, inflammation, and blood clotting. Aspirin belongs to the family of drugs called nonsteroidal anti-inflammatory agents. It is also being studied in cancer prevention. [NIH]

Assay: Determination of the amount of a particular constituent of a mixture, or of the biological or pharmacological potency of a drug. [EU]

Autologous: Taken from an individual's own tissues, cells, or DNA. [NIH]

Benign: Not cancerous; does not invade nearby tissue or spread to other parts of the body. [NIH]

Bereavement: Refers to the whole process of grieving and mourning and is associated with a deep sense of loss and sadness. [NIH]

Bevacizumab: A monoclonal antibody that may prevent the growth of blood vessels from surrounding tissue to a solid tumor. [NIH]

Bexarotene: An anticancer drug used to decrease the growth of some types of cancer cells. Also called LGD1069. [NIH]

Bilateral: Affecting both the right and left side of body. [NIH]

Bile: A fluid made by the liver and stored in the gallbladder. Bile is excreted into the small intestine where it helps digest fat. [NIH]

Biliary: Having to do with the liver, bile ducts, and/or gallbladder. [NIH]

Biochemical: Relating to biochemistry; characterized by, produced by, or involving chemical reactions in living organisms. [EU]

Biomarkers: Substances sometimes found in an increased amount in the blood, other body fluids, or tissues and that may suggest the presence of some types of cancer. Biomarkers include CA 125 (ovarian cancer), CA 15-3 (breast cancer), CEA (ovarian, lung, breast, pancreas, and GI tract cancers), and PSA (prostate cancer). Also called tumor markers. [NIH]

Biopsy: The removal of cells or tissues for examination under a microscope. When only a sample of tissue is removed, the procedure is called an incisional biopsy or core biopsy. When an entire tumor or lesion is removed, the procedure is called an excisional biopsy. When a sample of tissue or fluid is removed with a needle, the procedure is called a needle biopsy or fine-needle aspiration. [NIH]

Bladder: The organ that stores urine. [NIH]

Bleomycin: An anticancer drug that belongs to the family of drugs called antitumor antibiotics. [NIH]

Calcitonin: A hormone secreted by the thyroid that lowers blood calcium levels. [NIH]

Calcium: A mineral found in teeth, bones, and other body tissues. [NIH]

Carcinogenesis: The process by which normal cells are transformed into cancer cells. [NIH]

Carcinogenic: Producing carcinoma. [EU]

Carcinoma: Cancer that begins in the skin or in tissues that line or cover internal organs. [NIH]

Carcinosarcoma: A malignant tumor that is a mixture of carcinoma (cancer of epithelial tissue, which is skin and tissue that lines or covers the internal organs) and sarcoma (cancer of connective tissue, such as bone, cartilage, and fat). [NIH]

Catheter: A flexible tube used to deliver fluids into or withdraw fluids from the body. [NIH]

CEA: Carcinoembryonic antigen. A substance that is sometimes found in an increased amount in the blood of people with certain cancers. [NIH]

Cell: The individual unit that makes up all of the tissues of the body. All living things are made up of one or more cells. [NIH]

Cervical: Relating to the neck, or to the neck of any organ or structure. Cervical lymph nodes are located in the neck; cervical cancer refers to cancer of the uterine cervix, which is the lower, narrow end (the "neck") of the uterus. [NIH]

Cervix: The lower, narrow end of the uterus that forms a canal between the uterus and vagina. [NIH]

Charities: Social welfare organizations with programs designed to assist individuals in times of need. [NIH]

Chemotherapy: Treatment with anticancer drugs. [NIH]

Chlorambucil: An anticancer drug that belongs to the family of drugs called alkylating agents. [NIH]

Cholesterol: The principal sterol of all higher animals, distributed in body tissues, especially the brain and spinal cord, and in animal fats and oils. [NIH]

Chromosomal: Pertaining to chromosomes. [EU]

Chromosome: Part of a cell that contains genetic information. Except for sperm and eggs, all human cells contain 46 chromosomes. [NIH]

Chronic: A disease or condition that persists or progresses over a long period of time. [NIH]

Cisplatin: An anticancer drug that belongs to the family of drugs called platinum compounds. [NIH]

CNS: Central nervous system. The brain and spinal cord. [NIH]

Coenzyme: An organic nonprotein molecule, frequently a phosphorylated derivative of a water-soluble vitamin, that binds with the protein molecule (apoenzyme) to form the active enzyme (holoenzyme). [EU]

Collagen: A fibrous protein found in cartilage and other connective tissue. [NIH]

Constipation: Infrequent or difficult evacuation of the faeces. [EU]

Contamination: The soiling or pollution by inferior material, as by the introduction of organisms into a wound, or sewage into a stream. [EU]

Contraception: The prevention of conception or impregnation. [EU]

Corpus: The body of the uterus. [NIH]

Corticosteroids: Hormones that have antitumor activity in lymphomas and lymphoid leukemias; in addition, corticosteroids (steroids) may be used for hormone replacement and for the management of some of the complications of cancer and its treatment. [NIH]

Curative: Tending to overcome disease and promote recovery. [EU]

Cutaneous: Having to do with the skin. [NIH]

Cyclic: Pertaining to or occurring in a cycle or cycles; the term is applied to chemical compounds that contain a ring of atoms in the nucleus. [EU]

Cyclophosphamide: An anticancer drug that belongs to the family of drugs called alkylating agents. [NIH]

Cyclosporine: A drug used to help reduce the risk of rejection of organ and bone marrow transplants by the body. It is also used in clinical trials to make cancer cells more sensitive to anticancer drugs. [NIH]

Cystine: A covalently linked dimeric nonessential amino acid formed by the oxidation of cysteine. Two molecules of cysteine are joined together by a disulfide bridge to form cystine. [NIH]

Cytokines: A class of substances that are produced by cells of the immune system and can affect the immune response. Cytokines can also be produced in the laboratory by recombinant DNA technology and given to people to affect immune responses. [NIH]

Depsipeptide: Anticancer drugs obtained from microorganisms. [NIH]

Dermatitis: Inflammation of the skin. [NIH]

Dermatology: A medical specialty concerned with the skin, its structure, functions, diseases, and treatment. [NIH]

Diarrhea: Passage of excessively liquid or excessively frequent stools. [NIH]

Docetaxel: An anticancer drug that belongs to the family of drugs called mitotic inhibitors. [NIH]

Doxorubicin: An anticancer drug that belongs to the family of drugs called antitumor antibiotics. It is an anthracycline. [NIH]

Drosophila: A genus of small, two-winged flies containing approximately 900 described species. These organisms are the most extensively studied of all genera from the standpoint of genetics and cytology. [NIH]

Dysplasia: Cells that look abnormal under a microscope but are not cancer. [NIH]

Ectopic: Pertaining to or characterized by ectopia. [EU]

Elasticity: Resistance and recovery from distortion of shape. [NIH]

Encephalopathy: A disorder of the brain that can be caused by disease, injury, drugs, or chemicals. [NIH]

Endemic: Present or usually prevalent in a population or geographical area at all times; said of a disease or agent. Called also endemial. [EU]

Endocrinology: A subspecialty of internal medicine concerned with the metabolism, physiology, and disorders of the endocrine system. [NIH]

Endogenous: Produced inside an organism or cell. The opposite is external (exogenous) production. [NIH]

Endometrium: The layer of tissue that lines the uterus. [NIH]

Endoscopy: The use of a thin, lighted tube (called an endoscope) to examine the inside of the body. [NIH]

Epidemiological: Relating to, or involving epidemiology. [EU]

Epirubicin: An anticancer drug that belongs to the family of drugs called antitumor antibiotics. [NIH]

Epithelial: Refers to the cells that line the internal and external surfaces of the body. [NIH]

Epithelium: A thin layer of tissue that covers organs, glands, and other structures within the body. [NIH]

Esophageal: Having to do with the esophagus, the muscular tube through which food passes from the throat to the stomach. [NIH]

Esophagus: The muscular tube through which food passes from the throat to the stomach. [NIH]

Etoposide: An anticancer drug that is a podophyllotoxin derivative and belongs to the family of drugs called mitotic inhibitors. [NIH]

Exogenous: Developed or originating outside the organism, as exogenous disease. [EU]

Exons: Coding regions of messenger RNA included in the genetic transcript which survive the processing of RNA in cell nuclei to become part of a spliced messenger of structural RNA in the cytoplasm. They include joining and diversity exons of immunoglobulin genes. [NIH]

Extracorporeal: Situated or occurring outside the body. [EU]

Fibrosis: The growth of fibrous tissue. [NIH]

Filgrastim: A colony-stimulating factor that stimulates the production of neutrophils (a type of white blood cell). It is a cytokine that belongs to the family of drugs called hematopoietic (blood-forming) agents. Also called granulocyte colony-stimulating factor (G-CSF). [NIH]

Flavopiridol: Belongs to the family of anticancer drugs called flavinols. [NIH]

Fluorouracil: An anticancer drug that belongs to the family of drugs called antimetabolites. [NIH]

FR901228: An anticancer drug that belongs to the family of drugs called depsipeptides. [NIH]

Fractionation: Dividing the total dose of radiation therapy into several smaller, equal doses delivered over a period of several days. [NIH]

Gallium: A rare, metallic element designated by the symbol, Ga, atomic number 31, and atomic weight 69.72. [NIH]

Gastrointestinal: Refers to the stomach and intestines. [NIH]

Gene: The functional and physical unit of heredity passed from parent to offspring. Genes are pieces of DNA, and most genes contain the information for making a specific protein. [NIH]

Gland: An organ that produces and releases one or more substances for use in the body. Some glands produce fluids that affect tissues or organs. Others produce hormones or participate in blood production. [NIH]

Gliadin: Simple protein, one of the prolamines, derived from the gluten of wheat, rye, etc. May be separated into 4 discrete electrophoretic fractions. It is the toxic factor associated with celiac disease. [NIH]

Glioma: A cancer of the brain that comes from glial, or supportive, cells. [NIH]

Glucose: Sugar. [NIH]

Glutamine: An amino acid used in nutrition therapy. It is also being studied for the treatment of diarrhea caused by radiation therapy to the pelvis. [NIH]

Gluten: The protein of wheat and other grains which gives to the dough its tough elastic character. [EU]

Glycoprotein: A protein that has sugar molecules attached to it. [NIH]

Goiter: Enlargement of the thyroid gland. [NIH]

Grade: The grade of a tumor depends on how abnormal the cancer cells look under a microscope and how quickly the tumor is likely to grow and spread. Grading systems are different for each type of cancer. [NIH]

Graft: Healthy skin, bone, or other tissue taken from one part of the body and used to replace diseased or injured tissue removed from another part of the body. [NIH]

Grasses: A large family, gramineae, of narrow-leaved herbaceous monocots. Many grasses produce highly allergenic pollens and are hosts to cattle parasites and toxic fungi. [NIH]

Hematology: A subspecialty of internal medicine concerned with morphology, physiology, and pathology of the blood and blood-forming tissues. [NIH]

Histology: The study of tissues and cells under a microscope. [NIH]

Homeostasis: A tendency to stability in the normal body states (internal environment) of the organism. It is achieved by a system of control mechanisms activated by negative feedback; e.g. a high level of carbon dioxide in extracellular fluid triggers increased pulmonary ventilation, which in turn causes a decrease in carbon dioxide concentration. [EU]

Homologous: Corresponding in structure, position, origin, etc., as (a) the feathers of a bird and the scales of a fish, (b) antigen and its specific antibody, (c) allelic chromosomes. [EU]

Hormonal: Pertaining to or of the nature of a hormone. [EU]

Hormones: Chemicals produced by glands in the body and circulated in the bloodstream. Hormones control the actions of certain cells or organs. [NIH]

Hybridization: The genetic process of crossbreeding to produce a hybrid. Hybrid nucleic acids can be formed by nucleic acid hybridization of DNA and RNA molecules. Protein hybridization allows for hybrid proteins to be formed from polypeptide chains. [NIH]

Hyperplasia: An abnormal increase in the number of cells in an organ or tissue. [NIH]

Hypersecretion: Excessive secretion. [EU]

Hyperthyroidism: A condition in which the thyroid gland produces too much thyroid hormone. [NIH]

Hypothyroidism: Deficiency of thyroid activity. In adults, it is most common in women and is characterized by decrease in basal metabolic rate, tiredness and lethargy, sensitivity to cold, and menstrual disturbances. If untreated, it progresses to full-blown myxoedema. In infants, severe hypothyroidism leads to cretinism. In juveniles, the manifestations are intermediate, with less severe mental and developmental retardation and only mild symptoms of the adult form. When due to pituitary deficiency of thyrotropin secretion it is called secondary hypothyroidism. [EU]

Ifosfamide: An anticancer drug that belongs to the family of drugs called alkylating agents. [NIH]

Immunodeficiency: The decreased ability of the body to fight infection and disease. [NIH]

Immunotherapy: Treatment to stimulate or restore the ability of the immune system to fight infection and disease. Also used to lessen side effects that may be caused by some cancer treatments. Also called biological therapy or biological response modifier (BRM) therapy. [NIH]

Indicative: That indicates; that points out more or less exactly; that reveals fairly clearly. [EU]

Induction: The act or process of inducing or causing to occur, especially the production of a specific morphogenetic effect in the developing embryo through the influence of evocators or organizers, or the production of anaesthesia or unconsciousness by use of appropriate agents. [EU]

Infiltration: The diffusion or accumulation in a tissue or cells of substances not normal to it or in amounts of the normal. Also, the material so accumulated. [EU]

Infusion: A method of putting fluids, including drugs, into the bloodstream. Also called intravenous infusion. [NIH]

Inoperable: Not suitable to be operated upon. [EU]

Interferon: A biological response modifier (a substance that can improve the body's natural response to disease). Interferons interfere with the division of cancer cells and can slow tumor growth. There are several types of interferons, including interferon-alpha, -beta, and -gamma. These substances are normally produced by the body. They are also made in the laboratory for use in treating cancer and other diseases. [NIH]

Interphase: The interval between two successive cell divisions during which the chromosomes are not individually distinguishable and DNA replication occurs. [NIH]

Intraocular: Within the eye. [EU]

Intravenous: IV. Into a vein. [NIH]

Invasive: 1. having the quality of invasiveness. 2. involving puncture or incision of the skin or insertion of an instrument or foreign material into the body; said of diagnostic techniques. [EU]

Involution: 1. a rolling or turning inward. 2. one of the movements involved in the gastrulation of many animals. 3. a retrograde change of the entire body or in a particular organ, as the retrograde changes in the female genital organs that result in normal size after delivery. 4. the progressive degeneration occurring naturally with advancing age, resulting in shrivelling of organs or tissues. [EU]

Iodine: A nonmetallic element of the halogen group that is represented by the atomic symbol I, atomic number 53, and atomic weight of 126.90. It is a nutritionally essential element, especially important in thyroid hormone synthesis. In solution, it has anti-infective properties and is used topically. [NIH]

Ipsilateral: Having to do with the same side of the body. [NIH]

Irinotecan: An anticancer drug that belongs to a family of anticancer drugs called topoisomerase inhibitors. It is a camptothecin analogue. Also called CPT 11. [NIH]

Kinetic: Pertaining to or producing motion. [EU]

Lactation: The period of the secretion of milk. [EU]

Laryngoscope: A thin, lighted tube used to examine the larynx (voice box). [NIH]

Laryngoscopy: Examination of the larynx (voice box) with a mirror (indirect laryngoscopy) or with a laryngoscope (direct laryngoscopy). [NIH]

Larynx: The area of the throat containing the vocal cords and used for breathing, swallowing, and talking. Also called the voice box. [NIH]

Lesion: An area of abnormal tissue change. [NIH]

Leucovorin: A drug used to protect normal cells from high doses of the anticancer drug methotrexate. It is also used to increase the antitumor effects of fluorouracil and tegafur-uracil, an oral treatment alternative to intravenous fluorouracil. [NIH]

Leukemia: Cancer of blood-forming tissue. [NIH]

Levothyroxine: Levo isomer of the thyroid hormone thyroxine. It is used for replacement therapy in reduced or absent thyroid function. [NIH]

Lobe: A portion of an organ such as the liver, lung, breast, or brain. [NIH]

Lobectomy: The removal of a lobe. [NIH]

Localization: The process of determining or marking the location or site of a lesion or disease. May also refer to the process of keeping a lesion or disease in a specific location or site. [NIH]

Lubricants: Oily or slippery substances. [NIH]

Lymph: The almost colorless fluid that travels through the lymphatic system and carries cells that help fight infection and disease. [NIH]

Lymphadenopathy: Disease or swelling of the lymph nodes. [NIH]

Lymphocyte: A white blood cell. Lymphocytes have a number of roles in the immune system, including the production of antibodies and other substances that fight infection and diseases. [NIH]

Lymphocytic: Referring to lymphocytes, a type of white blood cell. [NIH]

Lymphoid: Referring to lymphocytes, a type of white blood cell. Also refers to tissue in which lymphocytes develop. [NIH]

Lymphoma: Cancer that arises in cells of the lymphatic system. [NIH]

Malignancy: A cancerous tumor that can invade and destroy nearby tissue and spread to other parts of the body. [NIH]

Malignant: Cancerous; a growth with a tendency to invade and destroy nearby tissue and spread to other parts of the body. [NIH]

Mammary: Pertaining to the mamma, or breast. [EU]

Mammogram: An x-ray of the breast. [NIH]

Mammography: The use of x-rays to create a picture of the breast. [NIH]

Medullary: Pertaining to the marrow or to any medulla; resembling marrow. [EU]

Melanoma: A form of skin cancer that arises in melanocytes, the cells that produce pigment. Melanoma usually begins in a mole. [NIH]

Membrane: A very thin layer of tissue that covers a surface. [NIH]

Mesothelioma: A benign (noncancerous) or malignant (cancerous) tumor affecting the lining of the chest or abdomen. Exposure to asbestos particles in the air increases the risk of developing malignant mesothelioma. [NIH]

Metaphase: The second phase of cell division, in which the chromosomes line up across the equatorial plane of the spindle prior to separation. [NIH]

Metastasis: The spread of cancer from one part of the body to another. Tumors formed from cells that have spread are called "secondary tumors" and contain cells that are like those in the original (primary) tumor. The plural is metastases. [NIH]

Metastasize: To spread from one part of the body to another. When cancer cells metastasize and form secondary tumors, the cells in the metastatic tumor are like those in the original (primary) tumor. [NIH]

Metastatic: Having to do with metastasis, which is the spread of cancer from one part of the body to another. [NIH]

Methoxsalen: A drug used in ultraviolet light therapy. [NIH]

Microscopy: The application of microscope magnification to the study of materials that cannot be properly seen by the unaided eye. [NIH]

Mitoguazone: Antineoplastic agent effective against myelogenous leukemia in experimental animals. Also acts as an inhibitor of animal S-adenosylmethionine decarboxylase. [NIH]

Mitoxantrone: An anticancer drug that belongs to the family of drugs called antitumor antibiotics. [NIH]

Molecular: Of, pertaining to, or composed of molecules : a very small mass of matter. [EU]

Molecule: A chemical made up of two or more atoms. The atoms in a molecule can be the same (an oxygen molecule has two oxygen atoms) or different (a water molecule has two hydrogen atoms and one oxygen atom). Biological molecules, such as proteins and DNA, can be made up of many thousands of atoms. [NIH]

Morphology: The science of the form and structure of organisms (plants, animals, and other forms of life). [NIH]

MRI: Magnetic resonance imaging (mag-NET-ik REZ-o- nans IM-a-jing). A procedure in which a magnet linked to a computer is used to create detailed pictures of areas inside the body. [NIH]

Mutagenesis: Process of generating genetic mutations. It may occur spontaneously or be induced by mutagens. [NIH]

Mycosis: Any disease caused by a fungus. [EU]

Myeloma: Cancer that arises in plasma cells, a type of white blood cell. [NIH]

Myxedema: A condition characterized by a dry, waxy type of swelling with abnormal deposits of mucin in the skin and other tissues. It is produced by a functional insufficiency of the thyroid gland, resulting in deficiency of thyroid hormone. The skin becomes puffy around the eyes and on the cheeks and the face is dull and expressionless with thickened nose and lips. The congenital form of the disease is cretinism. [NIH]

Nasopharynx: The upper part of the throat behind the nose. An opening on each side of the nasopharynx leads into the ear. [NIH]

Nausea: An unpleasant sensation, vaguely referred to the epigastrium and abdomen, and often culminating in vomiting. [EU]

Necrosis: Refers to the death of living tissues. [NIH]

Neonatal: Pertaining to the first four weeks after birth. [EU]

Neoplasm: A new growth of benign or malignant tissue. [NIH]

Neoplastic: Pertaining to or like a neoplasm (= any new and abnormal growth); pertaining to neoplasia (= the formation of a neoplasm). [EU]

Neural: 1. pertaining to a nerve or to the nerves. 2. situated in the region of the spinal axis, as the neutral arch. [EU]

Neuroendocrine: Having to do with the interactions between the nervous system and the endocrine system. Describes certain cells that release hormones into the blood in response to stimulation of the nervous system. [NIH]

Neurologic: Having to do with nerves or the nervous system. [NIH]

Neutropenia: An abnormal decrease in the number of neutrophils, a type of white blood cell. [NIH]

Neutrophil: A type of white blood cell. [NIH]

Occult: Obscure; concealed from observation, difficult to understand. [EU]

Ointments: Semisolid preparations used topically for protective emollient effects or as a vehicle for local administration of medications. Ointment bases are various mixtures of fats, waxes, animal and plant oils and solid and liquid hydrocarbons. [NIH]

Oncogene: A gene that normally directs cell growth. If altered, an oncogene can promote or allow the uncontrolled growth of cancer. Alterations can be inherited or caused by an environmental exposure to carcinogens. [NIH]

Oncologist: A doctor who specializes in treating cancer. Some oncologists specialize in a particular type of cancer treatment. For example, a radiation oncologist specializes in treating cancer with radiation. [NIH]

Oncology: The study of cancer. [NIH]

Oral: By or having to do with the mouth. [NIH]

Orthopaedic: Pertaining to the correction of deformities of the musculoskeletal system; pertaining to orthopaedics. [EU]

Osteoporosis: A condition that is characterized by a decrease in bone mass and density, causing bones to become fragile. [NIH]

Otolaryngology: A surgical specialty concerned with the study and treatment of disorders of the ear, nose, and throat. [NIH]

Ovary: Either of the paired glands in the female that produce the female germ cells and secrete some of the female sex hormones. [NIH]

Oxaliplatin: An anticancer drug that belongs to the family of drugs called platinum compounds. [NIH]

Paclitaxel: An anticancer drug that belongs to the family of drugs called mitotic inhibitors. [NIH]

Palliative: 1. affording relief, but not cure. 2. an alleviating medicine. [EU]

Pancreas: A glandular organ located in the abdomen. It makes pancreatic juices, which contain enzymes that aid in digestion, and it produces several hormones, including insulin. The pancreas is surrounded by the stomach, intestines, and other organs. [NIH]

Pancreatic: Having to do with the pancreas. [NIH]

Pap test: The collection of cells from the cervix for examination under a microscope. It is used to detect changes that may be cancer or may lead to cancer, and can show noncancerous conditions, such as infection or inflammation. Also called a Pap smear. [NIH]

Papillary: Pertaining to or resembling papilla, or nipple. [EU]

Papillomavirus: A genus of papovaviridae causing proliferation of the epithelium, which may lead to malignancy. A wide range of animals are infected including humans, chimpanzees, cattle, rabbits, dogs, and horses. [NIH]

Parathyroid: 1. situated beside the thyroid gland. 2. one of the parathyroid glands. 3. a sterile preparation of the water-soluble principle(s) of the parathyroid glands, ad-ministered parenterally as an antihypocalcaemic, especially in the treatment of acute hypoparathyroidism with tetany. [EU]

Pathologist: A doctor who identifies diseases by studying cells and tissues under a microscope. [NIH]

Pelvis: The lower part of the abdomen, located between the hip bones. [NIH]

Phenotype: The outward appearance of the individual. It is the product of interactions between genes and between the genotype and the environment. This includes the killer phenotype, characteristic of YEASTS. [NIH]

Phosphorylation: The introduction of a phosphoryl group into a compound through the formation of an ester bond between the compound and a phosphorus moiety. [NIH]

Plasma: The clear, yellowish, fluid part of the blood that carries the blood cells. The proteins that form blood clots are in plasma. [NIH]

Plasmacytoma: Cancer of the plasma cells (white blood cells that produce antibodies) that may turn into multiple myeloma. [NIH]

Platelets: A type of blood cell that helps prevent bleeding by causing blood clots to form. Also called thrombocytes. [NIH]

Polyposis: The development of numerous polyps (growths that protrude from a mucous membrane). [NIH]

Posterior: Situated in back of, or in the back part of, or affecting the back or dorsal surface of the body. In lower animals, it refers to the caudal end of the body. [EU]

Postoperative: After surgery. [NIH]

Potassium: A metallic element that is important in body functions such as regulation of blood pressure and of water content in cells, transmission of nerve impulses, digestion, muscle contraction, and heart beat. [NIH]

Preclinical: Before a disease becomes clinically recognizable. [EU]

Prednisolone: A synthetic corticosteroid used in the treatment of blood cell cancers (leukemias) and lymph system cancers (lymphomas). [NIH]

Prevalence: The total number of cases of a given disease in a specified population at a designated time. It is differentiated from incidence, which refers to the number of new cases in the population at a given time. [NIH]

Progression: Increase in the size of a tumor or spread of cancer in the body. [NIH]

Proline: A non-essential amino acid that is synthesized from glutamic acid. It is an essential component of collagen and is important for proper functioning of joints and tendons. [NIH]

Prostate: A gland in males that surrounds the neck of the bladder and the urethra. It secretes a substance that liquifies coagulated semen. It is situated in the pelvic cavity behind the lower part of the pubic symphysis, above the deep layer of the triangular ligament, and rests upon the rectum. [NIH]

Proteins: Polymers of amino acids linked by peptide bonds. The specific sequence of amino acids determines the shape and function of the protein. [NIH]

Psychotherapy: A generic term for the treatment of mental illness or emotional disturbances primarily by verbal or nonverbal communication. [NIH]

PTC: Percutaneous transhepatic cholangiography (per-kyoo-TAN-ee-us trans-heh-PAT-ik ko-LAN-jee-AH-gra-fee). A procedure to x-ray the bile ducts. In this procedure, a dye is injected through a thin needle inserted through the skin into the liver or the gallbladder, and an x-ray picture is taken. [NIH]

Radioimmunotherapy: Treatment with a radioactive substance that is linked to an antibody that will attach to the tumor when injected into the body. [NIH]

Radioisotope: An unstable element that releases radiation as it breaks down. Radioisotopes can be used in imaging tests or as a treatment for cancer. [NIH]

Radiolabeled: Any compound that has been joined with a radioactive substance. [NIH]

Radiology: The use of radiation (such as x-rays) or other imaging technologies (such as ultrasound and magnetic resonance imaging) to diagnose or treat disease. [NIH]

Radiotherapy: The treatment of disease by ionizing radiation. [EU]

Radium: Radium. A radioactive element of the alkaline earth series of metals. It has the atomic symbol Ra, atomic number 88, and atomic weight 226. Radium is the product of the disintegration of uranium and is present in pitchblende and all ores containing uranium. It is used clinically as a source of beta and gamma-rays in radiotherapy, particularly brachytherapy. [NIH]

Randomized: Describes an experiment or clinical trial in which animal or human subjects are assigned by chance to separate groups that compare different treatments. [NIH]

Receptor: A molecule inside or on the surface of a cell that binds to a specific substance and causes a specific physiologic effect in the cell. [NIH]

Recombinant: 1. a cell or an individual with a new combination of genes not found together in either parent; usually applied to linked genes. [EU]

Rectal: By or having to do with the rectum. The rectum is the last 8 to 10 inches of the large intestine and ends at the anus. [NIH]

Rectum: The last 8 to 10 inches of the large intestine. [NIH]

Recurrence: The return of cancer, at the same site as the original (primary) tumor or in another location, after the tumor had disappeared. [NIH]

Refractory: Not readily yielding to treatment. [EU]

Regimen: A treatment plan that specifies the dosage, the schedule, and the duration of treatment. [NIH]

Registries: The systems and processes involved in the establishment, support, management, and operation of registers, e.g., disease registers. [NIH]

Remission: A decrease in or disappearance of signs and symptoms of cancer. In partial remission, some, but not all, signs and symptoms of cancer have disappeared. In complete remission, all signs and symptoms of cancer have disappeared, although there still may be cancer in the body. [NIH]

Resection: Removal of tissue or part or all of an organ by surgery. [NIH]

Reserpine: An alkaloid found in the roots of Rauwolfia serpentina and R. vomitoria. Reserpine inhibits the uptake of norepinephrine into storage vesicles resulting in depletion of catecholamines and serotonin from central and peripheral axon terminals. It has been used as an antihypertensive and an antipsychotic as well as a research tool, but its adverse effects limit its clinical use. [NIH]

Retinoid: Vitamin A or a vitamin A-like compound. [NIH]

Retrospective: Looking back at events that have already taken place. [NIH]

Rheumatoid: Resembling rheumatism. [EU]

Rituximab: A type of monoclonal antibody used in cancer detection or therapy. Monoclonal antibodies are laboratory-produced substances that can locate and bind to cancer cells. [NIH]

Sarcoidosis: An idiopathic systemic inflammatory granulomatous disorder comprised of epithelioid and multinucleated giant cells with little necrosis. It usually invades the lungs with fibrosis and may also involve lymph nodes, skin, liver, spleen, eyes, phalangeal bones, and parotid glands. [NIH]

Sarcoma: A cancer of the bone, cartilage, fat, muscle, blood vessels or other connective or supportive tissue. [NIH]

Sargramostim: A colony-stimulating factor that stimulates the production of blood cells, especially platelets, during chemotherapy. It is a cytokine that belongs to the family of drugs called hematopoietic (blood-forming) agents. Also called GM-CSF. [NIH]

Screening: Checking for disease when there are no symptoms. [NIH]

Secretion: 1. the process of elaborating a specific product as a result of the activity of a gland; this activity may range from separating a specific substance of the blood to the elaboration of a new chemical substance. 2. any substance produced by secretion. [EU]

Sequela: Any lesion or affection following or caused by an attack of disease. [EU]

Serum: The clear liquid part of the blood that remains after blood cells and clotting proteins have been removed. [NIH]

Species: A taxonomic category subordinate to a genus (or subgenus) and superior to a subspecies or variety, composed of individuals possessing common characters distinguishing them from other categories of individuals of the same taxonomic level. In taxonomic nomenclature, species are designated by the genus name followed by a Latin or Latinized adjective or noun. [EU]

Sporadic: Neither endemic nor epidemic; occurring occasionally in a random or isolated manner. [EU]

Stabilization: The creation of a stable state. [EU]

Staging: Performing exams and tests to learn the extent of the cancer within the body, especially whether the disease has spread from the original site to other parts of the body. [NIH]

Steroid: A group name for lipids that contain a hydrogenated cyclopentanoperhydrophenanthrene ring system. Some of the substances included in this group are progesterone, adrenocortical hormones, the gonadal hormones, cardiac aglycones, bile acids, sterols (such as cholesterol), toad poisons, saponins, and some of the carcinogenic hydrocarbons. [EU]

Stomach: An organ that is part of the digestive system. It helps in the digestion of food by mixing it with digestive juices and churning it into a thin liquid. [NIH]

Supplementation: Adding nutrients to the diet. [NIH]

Suppressive: Tending to suppress : effecting suppression; specifically : serving to suppress activity, function, symptoms. [EU]

Symptomatic: Having to do with symptoms, which are signs of a condition or disease. [NIH]

Systemic: Affecting the entire body. [NIH]

Technetium: The first artificially produced element and a radioactive fission product of uranium. The stablest isotope has a mass number 99 and is used diagnostically as a radioactive imaging agent. Technetium has the atomic symbol Tc, atomic number 43, and atomic weight 98.91. [NIH]

Telomerase: Essential ribonucleoprotein reverse transcriptase that adds telomeric DNA to the ends of eukaryotic chromosomes. Telomerase appears to be repressed in normal human somatic tissues but reactivated in cancer, and thus may be necessary for malignant transformation. EC 2.7.7.-. [NIH]

Teniposide: An anticancer drug that is a podophyllotoxin derivative and belongs to the family of drugs called mitotic inhibitors. [NIH]

Teratoma: A type of germ cell tumor that may contain several different types of tissue, such as hair, muscle, and bone. Teratomas occur most often in the ovaries in women, the testicles in men, and the tailbone in children. Not all teratomas are malignant. [NIH]

Testis: Either of the paired male reproductive glands that produce the male germ cells and the male hormones. [NIH]

Thalidomide: A drug that belongs to the family of drugs called angiogenesis inhibitors. It prevents the growth of new blood vessels into a solid tumor. [NIH]

Thymus: An organ that is part of the lymphatic system, in which T lymphocytes grow and multiply. The thymus is in the chest behind the breastbone. [NIH]

Thyroid: A gland located near the windpipe (trachea) that produces thyroid hormone, which helps regulate growth and metabolism. [NIH]

Thyroid Hormones: Hormones secreted by the thyroid gland. [NIH]

Thyrotoxicosis: The condition resulting from presentation to the tissues of excessive quantities of the thyroid hormones, whether the excess results from overproduction by the thyroid gland (as in Graves' disease), originated outside the thyroid, or is due to loss of storage function and leakage from the gland. [EU]

Thyrotropin: A peptide hormone secreted by the anterior pituitary. It promotes the growth of the thyroid gland and stimulates the synthesis of thyroid hormones and the release of thyroxine by the thyroid gland. [NIH]

Tomography: A series of detailed pictures of areas inside the body; the pictures are created by a computer linked to an x-ray machine. [NIH]

Topotecan: An anticancer drug that belongs to the family drugs called topoisomerase inhibitors. [NIH]

Toxicity: The quality of being poisonous, especially the degree of virulence of a toxic microbe or of a poison. [EU]

Toxins: Poisons produced by certain animals, plants, or bacteria. [NIH]

Toxoplasmosis: An acute or chronic, widespread disease of animals and humans caused by the obligate intracellular protozoon Toxoplasma gondii, transmitted by oocysts containing the pathogen in the feces of cats (the definitive host), usually by contaminated soil, direct exposure to infected feces, tissue cysts in infected meat, or tachyzoites (proliferating forms) in blood. [EU]

Tracer: A substance (such as a radioisotope) used in imaging procedures. [NIH]

Tracheostomy: Surgery to create an opening (stoma) into the windpipe. The opening itself may also be called a tracheostomy. [NIH]

Transplantation: The replacement of an organ with one from another person. [NIH]

Tyrosine: A non-essential amino acid. In animals it is synthesized from phenylalanine. It is also the precursor of epinephrine, thyroid hormones, and melanin. [NIH]

Ultrasonography: A procedure in which sound waves (called ultrasound) are bounced off tissues and the echoes are converted to a picture (sonogram). [NIH]

Urine: Fluid containing water and waste products. Urine is made by the kidneys, stored in the bladder, and leaves the body through the urethra. [NIH]

Uterus: The small, hollow, pear-shaped organ in a woman's pelvis. This is the organ in which a fetus develops. Also called the womb. [NIH]

Uveitis: An inflammation of part or all of the uvea, the middle (vascular) tunic of the eye, and commonly involving the other tunics (the sclera and cornea, and the retina). [EU]

Vaccine: A substance or group of substances meant to cause the immune system to respond to a tumor or to microorganisms, such as bacteria or viruses. [NIH]

Vanadium: Vanadium. A metallic element with the atomic symbol V, atomic number 23, and atomic weight 50.94. It is used in the manufacture of vanadium steel. Prolonged exposure can lead to chronic intoxication caused by absorption usually via the lungs. [NIH]

Vascular: Pertaining to blood vessels or indicative of a copious blood supply. [EU]

Vertebral: Of or pertaining to a vertebra. [EU]

Vinblastine: An anticancer drug that belongs to the family of plant drugs called vinca alkaloids. It is a mitotic inhibitor. [NIH]

Vincristine: An anticancer drug that belongs to the family of plant drugs called vinca alkaloids. [NIH]

Vinorelbine: An anticancer drug that belongs to the family of plant drugs called vinca alkaloids. [NIH]

Withdrawal: 1. a pathological retreat from interpersonal contact and social involvement, as may occur in schizophrenia, depression, or schizoid avoidant and schizotypal personality disorders. 2. (DSM III-R) a substance-specific organic brain syndrome that follows the cessation of use or reduction in intake of a psychoactive substance that had been regularly used to induce a state of intoxication. [EU]

Xenograft: The cells of one species transplanted to another species. [NIH]

General Dictionaries and Glossaries

While the above glossary is essentially complete, the dictionaries listed here cover virtually all aspects of medicine, from basic words and phrases to more advanced terms (sorted alphabetically by title; hyperlinks provide rankings, information and reviews at Amazon.com):

- **The Cancer Dictionary** by Roberta Altman, Michael J., Md Sarg;
  Paperback - 368 pages, 2nd Revised edition (November 1999), Checkmark Books; ISBN: 0816039542;
  http://www.amazon.com/exec/obidos/ASIN/0816039542/icongroupinterna

- **Dictionary of Medical Acronymns & Abbreviations** by Stanley Jablonski (Editor), Paperback, 4th edition (2001), Lippincott Williams & Wilkins Publishers, ISBN: 1560534605,
  http://www.amazon.com/exec/obidos/ASIN/1560534605/icongroupinterna

- **Dictionary of Medical Terms : For the Nonmedical Person (Dictionary of Medical Terms for the Nonmedical Person, Ed 4)** by Mikel A. Rothenberg, M.D, et al, Paperback - 544 pages, 4th edition (2000), Barrons Educational Series, ISBN: 0764112015,
http://www.amazon.com/exec/obidos/ASIN/0764112015/icongroupinterna

- **A Dictionary of the History of Medicine** by A. Sebastian, CD-Rom edition (2001), CRC Press-Parthenon Publishers, ISBN: 185070368X,
http://www.amazon.com/exec/obidos/ASIN/185070368X/icongroupinterna

- **Dorland's Illustrated Medical Dictionary (Standard Version)** by Dorland, et al, Hardcover - 2088 pages, 29th edition (2000), W B Saunders Co, ISBN: 0721662544,
http://www.amazon.com/exec/obidos/ASIN/0721662544/icongroupinterna

- **Dorland's Electronic Medical Dictionary** by Dorland, et al, Software, 29th Book & CD-Rom edition (2000), Harcourt Health Sciences, ISBN: 0721694934,
http://www.amazon.com/exec/obidos/ASIN/0721694934/icongroupinterna

- **Dorland's Pocket Medical Dictionary (Dorland's Pocket Medical Dictionary, 26th Ed)** Hardcover - 912 pages, 26th edition (2001), W B Saunders Co, ISBN: 0721682812,
http://www.amazon.com/exec/obidos/ASIN/0721682812/icongroupinterna/103-4193558-7304618

- **Melloni's Illustrated Medical Dictionary (Melloni's Illustrated Medical Dictionary, 4th Ed)** by Melloni, Hardcover, 4th edition (2001), CRC Press-Parthenon Publishers, ISBN: 85070094X,
http://www.amazon.com/exec/obidos/ASIN/85070094X/icongroupinterna

- **Stedman's Electronic Medical Dictionary Version 5.0 (CD-ROM for Windows and Macintosh, Individual)** by Stedmans, CD-ROM edition (2000), Lippincott Williams & Wilkins Publishers, ISBN: 0781726328,
http://www.amazon.com/exec/obidos/ASIN/0781726328/icongroupinterna

- **Stedman's Medical Dictionary** by Thomas Lathrop Stedman, Hardcover - 2098 pages, 27th edition (2000), Lippincott, Williams & Wilkins, ISBN: 068340007X,
http://www.amazon.com/exec/obidos/ASIN/068340007X/icongroupinterna

- **Stedman's Oncology Words** by Beverly J. Wolpert (Editor), Stedmans; Paperback - 502 pages, 3rd edition (June 15, 2000), Lippincott, Williams & Wilkins; ISBN: 0781726549;
http://www.amazon.com/exec/obidos/ASIN/0781726549/icongroupinterna

- **Tabers Cyclopedic Medical Dictionary (Thumb Index)** by Donald Venes (Editor), et al, Hardcover - 2439 pages, 19th edition (2001), F A Davis Co.,

ISBN: 0803606540,
http://www.amazon.com/exec/obidos/ASIN/0803606540/icongroupinterna

INDEX

A
Abdomen......70, 113, 125, 142, 266, 268, 269
Acne...146
Adenocarcinoma 128
Adenoma...80
Adenosine 91, 110, 257
Adenovirus.......................................83
Agonists...87
Amifostine............................... 214, 215
Amyloidosis 140, 257
Anaplastic...... 12, 14, 79, 107, 144, 147, 153, 155, 158, 164, 210, 216
Angiogenesis............... 70, 140, 258, 273
Antibody ...68, 70, 92, 112, 247, 248, 258, 263, 270, 272
Antigen...... 68, 110, 112, 212, 258, 259, 263
Aplidine 132
Apoptosis 85, 210, 215
Aspiration 26, 90, 107, 108, 162, 210, 259
Assay 86, 97
Autologous 216

B
Benign.. 4, 79, 80, 99, 102, 105, 109, 113, 145, 146, 152, 266, 268
Bereavement 36
Bilateral 148, 152, 163
Bile.......... 70, 83, 114, 124, 259, 270, 273
Biochemical............................... 88, 152
Biopsy..... 12, 26, 90, 106, 107, 162, 254, 259
Bladder...............................70, 118, 274

C
Calcitonin 108, 152, 153, 162, 253
Calcium........................... 83, 110, 259
Carcinogenesis..................................78
Carcinogenic.............................. 70, 273
Carcinosarcoma 147
Cervical 35, 47, 97, 107, 109, 145, 147, 148, 150, 151, 244, 260
Cervix.......................... 47, 118, 260, 269
Chemotherapy 18, 37, 52, 59, 70, 81, 163, 164, 165, 207, 209, 210, 213, 247, 257, 272
Chlorambucil.....................................52
Cholesterol 70, 83, 273
Chromosomal 78
Chronic........173, 178, 234, 249, 274, 275
Cisplatin 160, 161, 163, 164, 165
Contamination 215
Contraception 119
Corpus 168
Corticosteroids 68, 260
Curative 37, 160, 161
Cutaneous 138
Cyclic..91
Cyclophosphamide..........................163
Cystine........................... 88, 111, 261
Cytokines 101

D
Diarrhea 141, 263
Doxorubicin 160, 161, 163, 164, 165

E
Ectopic..106
Endemic........................... 115, 120, 272
Endocrinology...........................145, 146
Endogenous 87
Epidemiological............................ 79, 82
Epirubicin 94
Epithelial 81, 177, 259
Epithelium 83, 178, 269
Esophageal 84
Esophagus 111, 118, 262
Etoposide 213
Exogenous 111, 154, 155, 156, 157, 158, 159, 177, 261, 262
Exons.................................. 85, 111, 262

F
Fibrosis 142, 272
Fluorouracil 163, 200, 211, 266

G
Gene.... 12, 78, 79, 81, 83, 84, 85, 87, 88, 91, 96, 97, 105, 107, 110, 113, 118, 145, 153, 162, 175, 257, 268
Gluten 141, 263
Glycoprotein 88
Goiter..............86, 88, 102, 120, 123, 146
Grade..52, 69, 263
Grasses 141, 263

H
Histology 145
Homologous 88
Hormonal 133, 152
Hormones 11, 15, 16, 26, 70, 88, 113, 114, 123, 125, 263, 268, 269, 273
Hyperplasia 130, 152, 162
Hypersecretion 123
Hyperthyroidism.................................23
Hypothyroidism.....................23, 26, 264

I

Indicative 123, 142, 275
Induction...86
Infiltration..210
Infusion 69, 84, 216, 264
Inoperable 207
Interferon 69, 265
Intravenous 59, 69, 200, 264, 266
Invasive..................................... 80, 191
Involution..86
Iodine 15, 16, 17, 18, 19, 87, 97, 100, 101, 104, 119, 128, 134, 163, 165, 214, 215, 216
Ipsilateral... 148

L

Lactation..83
Laryngoscope 265
Laryngoscopy 265
Larynx 4, 112, 265
Lesion 26, 112, 130, 259, 266, 272
Leukemia..................... 27, 168, 173, 267
Lobe................. 16, 17, 27, 156, 159, 266
Lobectomy..... 16, 17, 106, 154, 155, 156, 157, 158, 159
Localization............................84, 87, 91
Lymphadenopathy 162
Lymphocyte 248, 258
Lymphoid................................... 68, 260
Lymphoma....52, 118, 138, 147, 153, 168, 173, 210, 212, 213, 214

M

Malignancy 144, 163, 178, 269
Malignant....... 4, 11, 79, 84, 89, 113, 115, 145, 152, 153, 173, 177, 178, 259, 266, 268, 273
Mammary 86
Mammography 34
Medullary....12, 90, 92, 93, 108, 130, 144, 146, 151, 152, 153, 162, 163, 209, 212
Melanoma...................... 76, 84, 168, 173
Membrane 81, 84, 178, 270
Mesothelioma 84, 113, 266
Metastasis....81, 107, 113, 146, 147, 148, 152, 163, 164, 215, 267
Metastasize 144, 151, 177, 267
Metastatic...... 81, 99, 103, 104, 163, 177, 209, 212, 214, 267
Microscopy 78
Molecular...80, 82, 83, 103, 166, 170, 172
Molecule 114, 142, 247, 248, 258, 260, 267, 271
Morphology 102, 141, 263
Mutagenesis 88
Myeloma................................76, 248, 269
Myxedema 123

N

Nasopharynx 118, 125, 268
Nausea 207
Necrosis...........................96, 142, 272
Neoplasm 4, 113, 268
Neoplastic 79, 212
Neural 79, 83

O

Occult 152
Oncogene 113, 133, 162, 173, 268
Oncologist................................. 47, 268
Oncology..................................... 21, 82
Oral...200, 266
Osteoporosis 128
Ovary 76, 118

P

Paclitaxel...............................210, 216
Palliative 37, 82
Pancreas......68, 114, 118, 125, 248, 257, 259, 269
Pancreatic.....89, 125, 168, 173, 207, 269
Parathyroid...79, 114, 120, 128, 152, 162, 269
Pelvis 125, 141, 168, 263, 274
Phenotype 114, 269
Phosphorylation.................................85
Plasma............70, 86, 113, 248, 267, 269
Plasmacytoma 213
Platelets 70, 272
Posterior... 130
Postoperative 145, 154, 155, 156, 157, 159
Potassium 25
Preclinical...................................... 192
Prevalence 78
Progression 80, 81, 153
Prostate . 37, 76, 118, 168, 173, 201, 206, 207, 248, 259
Proteins.. 70, 91, 112, 115, 142, 193, 247, 258, 264, 267, 269, 272
Psychotherapy 201, 206

R

Radioactive 15, 17, 18, 19, 70, 81, 87, 97, 100, 104, 115, 129, 134, 165, 214, 248, 270, 271, 273
Radioimmunotherapy 209, 212
Radioisotope 116, 274
Radiotherapy 108, 145, 146, 165, 210, 248, 271
Randomized 160, 161, 163, 164, 165
Receptor 84, 86, 88, 92, 101, 211, 248, 258
Recombinant 80, 83, 88, 91, 100, 109, 111, 261
Rectal 168
Rectum 118, 178, 271

Recurrence...... 132, 135, 144, 145, 154, 155, 156, 157, 159, 164
Regimen 163
Registries 98, 118
Remission.................... 97, 115, 164, 271
Resection 82, 144, 153, 154, 157, 164
Reserpine...210
Retinoid 87
Retrospective.......................... 144, 146
Rheumatoid 83, 212

S
Sarcoma........................... 147, 177, 259
Screening ...37, 56, 58, 61, 135, 152, 153, 162
Secretion 26, 88, 112, 115, 125, 264, 265, 272
Sequela 129
Serum 79, 92, 94, 97, 145, 216
Species .. 68, 88, 111, 115, 116, 257, 261, 272, 275
Sporadic 105, 152, 153, 162
Stabilization 85
Staging 12, 14, 92, 106, 147, 151, 153
Stomach.......68, 111, 118, 124, 125, 141, 168, 257, 262, 269
Supplementation 83, 212
Symptomatic..................................... 163
Systemic......... 16, 81, 140, 142, 257, 272

T
Technetium 101
Telomerase 95
Teratoma... 146
Thymus 146, 178, 273
Thyroid Hormones 115, 116, 274
Thyrotropin 26, 88, 94, 100, 104, 109, 264
Tomography 93, 104
Topotecan 83
Toxicity...................................... 86, 103
Toxins 88, 247, 258
Tracer 91, 129
Tracheostomy........................ 19, 27, 274
Tyrosine 211

U
Ultrasonography 95
Urine............................68, 124, 258, 259
Uterus 47, 118, 124, 177, 260, 261

V
Vanadium 249, 275
Vascular 144, 145, 151, 249, 274
Vertebral 134
Vinblastine...................................... 211
Vincristine 163

W
Withdrawal 91, 135

X
Xenograft 81